Self-Assessment Color Review
# Rabbit Medicine and Surgery
## Second Edition

T0321318

Self-Assessment Color Review

# Rabbit Medicine and Surgery

## Second Edition

### Emma Keeble
BVSc, DZooMed,
RCVS Recognised Specialist in Zoo and Wildlife Medicine, MRCVS
Clinician in Rabbit, Exotic Animal and Wildlife Medicine and Surgery
Royal (Dick) School of Veterinary Studies, The University of Edinburgh,
Easter Bush Veterinary Centre

### Anna Meredith
MA VetMB, PhD, CertLAS DZooMed, DipECZM MRCVS,
Professor of Zoological and Conservation Medicine
Director of Postgraduate Taught Programmes
Royal (Dick) School of Veterinary Studies, The University of Edinburgh,
Easter Bush Veterinary Centre

### Jenna Richardson
BVM&S MRCVS
Clinician in Rabbit, Exotic Animal and Wildlife Medicine and Surgery
Royal (Dick) School of Veterinary Studies, The University of Edinburgh,
Easter Bush Veterinary Centre

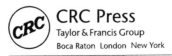

**CRC Press**
Taylor & Francis Group
Boca Raton  London  New York

CRC Press is an imprint of the
Taylor & Francis Group, an **informa** business

CRC Press
Taylor & Francis Group
6000 Broken Sound Parkway NW, Suite 300
Boca Raton, FL 33487-2742

© 2016 by Taylor & Francis Group, LLC
CRC Press is an imprint of Taylor & Francis Group, an Informa business

No claim to original U.S. Government works

Printed on acid-free paper
Version Date: 20160208

International Standard Book Number-13: 978-1-4987-3079-2 (Paperback)

**Visit the Taylor & Francis Web site at**
**http://www.taylorandfrancis.com**

**and the CRC Press Web site at**
**http://www.crcpress.com**

# Picture Acknowledgements

The editors gratefully acknowledge colleagues listed below who contributed illustrations for use in this book:

2a, 2b and 22 reproduced from the *Manual of Rabbit Medicine and Surgery*, edited by Paul A Fleckness (2000), with permissions of the BSAVA.

15a courtesy of Liam Reid.

15b and 112 courtesy of David Perpiñan.

23 and 78 courtesy of Fur and Feathers Magazine (www.furandfeather.co.uk)

63a and 63b courtesy of Natalie Antinoff.

70 and 87 reproduced from the *Manual of Rabbit medicine and Surgery*, edited by Paul A Fleckness (2000), with permission of R Harvey and the BSAVA.

107 courtesy of David Crossley.

112 courtesy of David Perpiñán.

143 courtesy of Neil McIntyre.

148a, 148b and 196 courtesy of Ron Rees Davies.

150a reproduced from White SD, Linder K, Shultheiss P *et al* (2000). Sebaceous adenitis in four rabbits (*Oryctologus caniculus*). *Veterinary Dermatology* 11: 53–61, with permission of Blackwell Publishing.

190 and 192 courtesy of Kevin Eatwell.

194 courtesty of LAVA.

# Preface

The relationship between rabbits and man goes back over more than 3000 years and continues to the present day. Today, rabbits are commonly kept as companion animals and are now increasingly popular pets for both children and adults, often being kept as 'house rabbits' indoors as a member of the family. Our understanding of a pet rabbit's physical and behavioural needs has made important advances since the first edition of the book was published, and this is reflected in this new edition. Rabbits are intelligent animals with husbandry requirements for adequate space, exercise, companionship and environmental stimulation. Better understanding of a rabbit's dietary needs has led to an improved quality of life for pet rabbits, improved commercial diets and greater awareness of the pathogenesis and treatment of rabbit dental disease. There is still, however, a real need for further research into these subject areas to develop a better veterinary understanding and to improve client education. We hope that this book will encourage those who read it towards this goal.

The expectation for high quality veterinary care of pet rabbits continues to drive great advancements in the field of rabbit medicine and surgery. This is a rapidly expanding area of veterinary practice, and there are increasing numbers of information sources available to veterinary personnel. This book is unique among those sources in that it is a practical, easy-to-read, photographic illustrated reference book, extremely useful both in a clinical situation to help diagnose and treat a clinical case and also as a revision source or test of knowledge for those taking graduate or postgraduate examinations in exotic animal medicine.

This book is designed to cover all major categories of rabbit medicine and surgery from basic biology and husbandry to more advanced diagnostic, medical and surgical techniques. In the new edition there is an increased emphasis on diagnostic and imaging techniques, as well as recent advances in emergency care, analgesia and rabbit surgery. All the questions have been updated, with the addition of many new illustrations, and new questions have also been added. This is not intended to be a comprehensive text, and no references are given. We have drawn on our own experience and the expertise of experienced rabbit clinicians to provide a wide range of cases and scenarios. In some cases the answers will not be definitive but will be based on the personal experience and opinion of the author. Drugs, where listed, are defined by their generic name and may not be available in all countries. It should also be noted that few drugs are licensed for use in pet rabbits, and there will be country-specific legislation governing the prescription of drugs for this species by veterinary surgeons.

We hope that readers will find this book informative as well as an enjoyable means of learning new facts, modifying their clinical approach to cases and consolidating their existing knowledge.

Emma Keeble
Anna Meredith
Jenna Richardson

# Acknowledgements

We would like to thank Jill Northcott and CRC Press for commissioning a revision of this book, all the contributors for giving up their time and sharing their expertise, and our families for their continued support.

# Contributors

**Wendy Bament** RVN, MSc, BSc(hons), CertVNES
The Veterinary Department
Marwell Wildlife (Zoological Park)
Winchester, UK

**Ian P. Boydell** BVetMed CertVOphthal MRCVS
Animal Medical Centre Referral Services
Manchester, UK

**Jeleen Briscoe** VMD
Matthew J Ryan Veterinary Hospital
of the University of Pennsylvania
Philadelphia, PA, USA

**Michelle L. Campbell-Ward**
BVSc(Hons I) DZooMed(Mammalian)
MANZCVS (Zoo Medicine) MRCVS
RCVS Recognised Specialist in Zoo
and Wildlife Medicine Veterinarian
Taronga Conservation Society Australia
Taronga Western Plains Zoo - Wildlife
Hospital, Australia

**Kevin Eatwell** BVSc (hons)
DZooMed (Reptilian) DipECZM
(Herpetological and Small Mammals)
MRCVS
Senior Lecturer in Exotic Animal and
Wildlife Medicine
The Royal (Dick) School of Veterinary
Studies
The University of Edinburgh
Easter Bush Veterinary Centre, UK

**Phillip P. Elliot** BVM&S MSC MRCVS
Small World Vet Centre
Hampshire, UK

**Jo Hedley** BVM&S DZooMed
(Reptilian) DipECZM (Herpetology)
MRCVS
Lecturer in Exotic Species and Small
Mammal Medicine and Surgery
RVC Exotics Service
Royal Veterinary College
London, UK

**Emma J. Keeble** BVSc DZooMed
RCVS Recognised Specialist in Zoo
and Wildlife Medicine, MRCVS
Clinician in Rabbit, Exotic
Animal and Wildlife Medicine and
Surgery
Royal (Dick) School of Veterinary
Studies, The University of Edinburgh
Easter Bush Veterinary Centre, UK

**Angela M. Lennox** DVM, Dipl ABVP-
Avian, Exotic Companion Mammal
Dipl ECZM-Small Mammals
Avian and Exotic Animal Clinic of
Indianapolis
Indianapolis, USA

**Emma Lightfoot** BVSc (Zoo), MA
(Applied Animal Behaviour and
Welfare)
Ipswich, Suffolk, UK

**Brigitte Lord** BVetMed(Hons)
CertZooMed MRCVS
The Royal (Dick) School of Veterinary
Studies
The University of Edinburgh
Easter Bush Veterinary Centre, UK

**Elizabeth Mancinelli** DVM
CertZooMed ECZM Dipl
(Small Mammal)
European Veterinary Specialist
Zoological Medicine MRCVS
Bath Referrals, Rosemary Lodge
Veterinary Hospital, Bath, UK

**Anna L. Meredith** MA VetMB PhD
CertLAS DZooMed DipECZM
MRCVS
Professor of Zoological and
Conservation Medicine
Director of Postgraduate Taught
Programmes
Royal (Dick) School of Veterinary
Studies, The University of Edinburgh
Easter Bush Veterinary Centre, UK

**David Perpiñán** DVM, MSc, Dip
ECZM (Herpetology)
Lecturer in Exotic Animal and
Wildlife Medicine
Hospital for Small Animals,
The Royal (Dick) School of
Veterinary Studies, The University
of Edinburgh, UK

**Romain Pizzi** BVSc MSc DZooMed
MACVSc(Surg) FRES FRGS MRCVS
Veterinary Surgeon, Zoological
Society of Scotland, Edinburgh Zoo,
Edinburgh, UK

**Jenna Richardson** BVM&S MRCVS
Clinician in Rabbit, Exotic
Animal and Wildlife Medicine and
Surgery
Royal (Dick) School of Veterinary
Studies, The University of Edinburgh
Easter Bush Veterinary Centre, UK

**Karen L. Rosenthal** DVM MS
ABVP(Avian)
Dean, School of Veterinary Medicine
St. Matthew's University
Cayman Islands, B.W.I.

**Lesa Thompson** MA BVM&S
DZooMed MSc MRCVS
Toxicology Laboratory
Department of Environmental
Veterinary Sciences
Graduate School of Veterinary
Medicine
Hokkaido University
Sapporo, Japan

# Abbreviations

| | | | |
|---|---|---|---|
| AIPMMA | antibiotic-impregnated polymethylmethacrylate (beads) | i/m | intramuscular |
| | | i/p | intraperitoneal |
| | | i/v | intravenous |
| ALP | alkaline phosphatase | LDH | lactate dehydrogenase |
| ALT | alanine aminotransferase | LH | luteinizing hormone |
| APP | acute phase protein | MCHC | mean cell haemoglobin concentration |
| APR | acute phase response | | |
| ARF | acute renal failure | MCV | mean corpuscular volume |
| AST | aspartate aminotransferase | MRI | magnetic resonance imaging |
| BP | blood pressure | | |
| bpm | beats per minute | NSAID | non-steroidal anti-inflammatory drug |
| BUN | blood urea nitrogen | | |
| CAR | cilia-associated respiratory (bacillus) | PCR | polymerase chain reaction |
| | | PCV | packed cell volume |
| CK | creatine kinase | PECA | partial ear canal ablation |
| CN | cranial nerve | PM | postmortem |
| CNS | central nervous system | PMMA | polymethylmethacrylate (beads) |
| CPK | creatine phosphokinase | | |
| CRP | C-reactive protein | p/o | *per os* (by mouth) |
| CSF | cerebrospinal fluid | RBCs | red blood cells |
| CT | computed tomography | RHD | rabbit haemorrhagic disease |
| DIC | disseminated intravascular coagulation | | |
| | | RHDV | rabbit haemorrhagic disease virus |
| EDTA | ethylenediamine tetra-acetic acid | | |
| | | rpm | revolutions per minute |
| ELISA | enzyme-linked immunosorbent assay | s/c | subcutaneous |
| | | SG | specific gravity |
| ERE | epizootic rabbit enteropathy (enterocolitis) | TECA | total ear canal ablation |
| | | TP | total protein |
| FSH | follicle-stimulating hormone | UK | United Kingdom |
| | | UPC | urinary protein:creatinine ratio |
| GGT | gamma glutamyltransferase | | |
| GI | gastrointestinal | USA | United States of America |
| Hb | haemoglobin | WBCs | white blood cells |
| Ig | immunoglobulin (antibody) | | |

# Classification of Cases

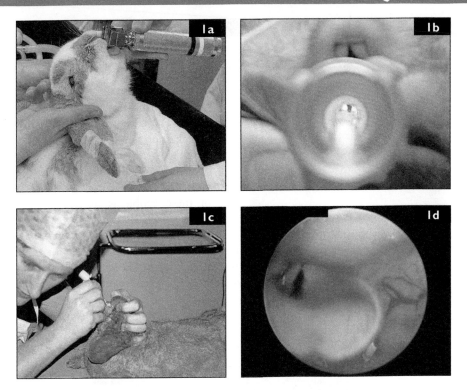

**CASE 1** Describe the techniques available for endotracheal intubation of an anaesthetized rabbit (**1a, b, c, d**).

**CASE 2** A 5-month-old New Zealand White rabbit is presented with a history of sudden onset blindness noticed when it was moved from a hutch to a much larger enclosed grass area. On clinical examination the globes are slightly larger (buphthalmia) than those of its companions.

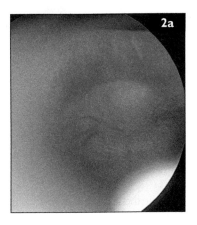

1  Describe what can be seen (**2a**).
2  What is the prognosis in this case?

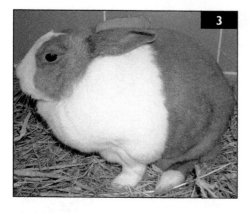

CASE 3 This 4-year-old female neutered house rabbit (3) has been hospitalized for assessment and treatment of a chronic GI hypomotility problem and a more recent perineal accumulation of uneaten caecotrophs. Clinical examination and diagnostic tests have led to the conclusion that obesity is a significant contributory factor in the development of both of these problems in this patient. A review of the history reveals that the diet consists of a mixed ration (muesli) concentrate provided *ad libitum*, a handful of yoghurt/carob drops each morning, occasional fresh greens or table scraps and access to a small amount of hay twice a week. The rabbit is housed in an indoor run and is let out into the living area at weekends to interact with the children.

1 What is the definition of obesity?
2 How would you achieve weight loss in this rabbit?

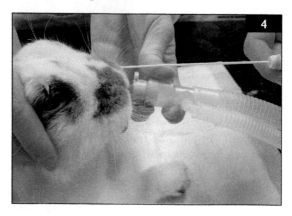

CASE 4 A deep nasal swab is being obtained in this rabbit for bacterial and fungal culture (4).

1 Describe how this is performed.
2 What alternative method could be employed?
3 What is the significance of a mixed bacterial culture being obtained?

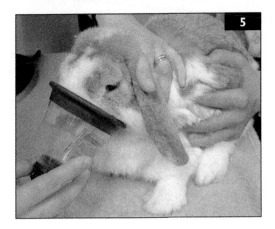

**CASE 5** Why is mask induction with a volatile anaesthetic agent risky in an unsedated rabbit (5)?

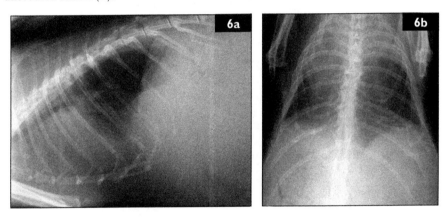

**CASE 6** A 7-year-old intact male English rabbit, housed indoors, presents with acute onset tachypnoea and laboured breathing. There is a 3-month history of weight loss, hindlimb weakness and rapid fatigue. The rabbit is alert, thin and weak. The mucous membranes are pale, with prolonged capillary refill time. A good response is noted to oxygen administration. The rabbit is sedated with intravenous midazolam and lateral and ventrodorsal radiographs of the thorax are taken (6a, b).

1 What are the differential diagnoses in this case?
2 Based on the radiographic findings, what immediate treatment would you consider?
3 What further diagnostic tests might be helpful?

**CASE 7** A 4-month-old male Dwarf Lop rabbit living outside in a hutch is destructive each time it comes into the home. The owners also report that the rabbit uses a litter tray in the home but leaves faecal pellets on the carpet from time to time. Ideally, the owners would like to bring it into the home but they are concerned by its behaviour. The rabbit is fed on a diet of concentrated food plus small amounts of hay and lots of fresh fruit and vegetables. What advice would you give the owners regarding this destructive behaviour?

**CASE 8** A 6-year-old castrated male crossbred rabbit is presented with chronic weight loss, decreased appetite and lethargy. An oral examination and skull radiographs show no evidence of dental disease. Blood is taken. In-house serum biochemistry analysis and haematology performed at an external laboratory yields the following results:

|  | SI units | Range |
|---|---|---|
| RBCs | $3.70 \times 10^{12}/l$* | (4.8–7.2) |
| Hb | $45 \times g/l$* | (103–155) |
| PCV | 0.17 l/l* | (0.35–0.48) |
| MCV | 46.7 fl* | (61–76) |
| MCHC | $260 \times g/l$* | (282–342) |
| WBCs | $1.2 \times 10^9/l$* | (3.3–12.0) |
| Neutrophils | $0.89 \times 10^9/l$* | (2.6–6.0) |
| Lymphocytes | $0.29 \times 10^9/l$* | (1.8–6.3) |
| Monocytes | $0.02 \times 10^9/l$ | (0–1.8) |
| Albumin | 19 g/l* | (35.9–41.4) |
| ALT | 51 iu/l | (22.1–80.2) |
| TP | 46 g/l* | (53–79) |
| Urea | 17.3 mmol/l* | (3.0–9.5) |
| * indicates result outside reference range. | | |

1 What are the main abnormalities?
2 What is the likely cause?
3 How may this be confirmed?

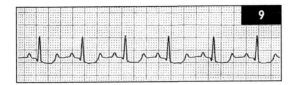

**CASE 9** A trace from lead II of the electrocardiogram of the rabbit in case 6 is shown (9). The echocardiogram revealed biatrial enlargement and evidence suggesting reduced systolic function. The rabbit was normotensive and the haematology and serum biochemistry results were unremarkable.

1 Describe the findings shown by lead II of the electrocardiogram.
2 What treatment is indicated?
3 What is the prognosis?

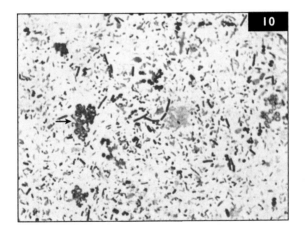

**CASE 10** A Gram-stained faecal smear from a 6-week-old male New Zealand White rabbit that presented with peracute onset diarrhoea, anorexia and depression is shown (10).

1 Identify the indicated organism. Why is this staining not what one would expect?
2 Is this organism a normal part of the rabbit enteric flora?
3 What specific requirements are needed for isolating this organism?
4 What causes the clinical signs seen?
5 What factors predispose to the development of clostridial enterotoxaemia?

## CASE 11

1 What are the potential benefits of spaying does, and what is the recommended age for this procedure?
2 Describe the surgical technique of ovariohysterectomy in the rabbit.
3 Are there any alternatives to surgical ovariohysterectomy?

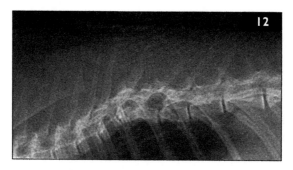

**CASE 12** A 6-month-old rabbit presents with a recent history of progressive hindlimb weakness. A lateral radiograph is taken (**12**).

1 What is the lesion shown?
2 What surgical treatment option is available?

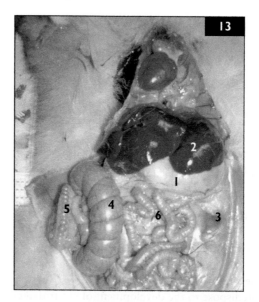

**CASE 13** Identify the organs labelled 1–6 on this rabbit abdomen (**13**).

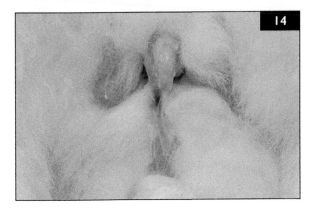

**CASE 14** Describe placement of a urethral catheter to obtain a urine sample in a buck rabbit (**14**).

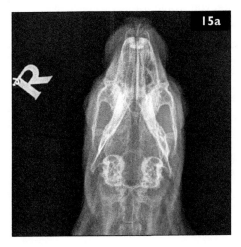

**CASE 15** A 5-year-old neutered female rabbit presented as a referral for a 4-year history of ongoing sneezing and purulent nasal discharge, particularly from the right nostril. The condition had been treated on several occasions with trimethoprim-sulfamethoxazole, with little to moderate response. Recently, a culture from the nasal discharge yielded growth of *Pasteurella multocida* (sensitive to trimethoprim-sulfamethoxazole) and a dorsoventral skull radiograph was taken (**15a**).

1  What are the radiographic findings?
2  What additional diagnostic tests can be performed to better define the problem?
3  How would you treat this case?

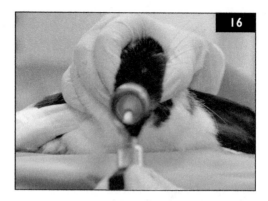

**CASE 16** On routine clinical examination of a pet rabbit you wish to perform a conscious examination of the oral cavity (**16**).

1  Describe the method you would use.
2  Can an accurate dental assessment be made?

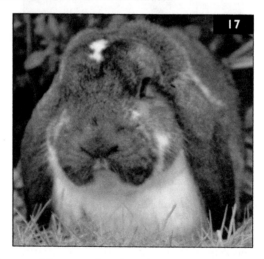

**CASE 17** A 2-year-old entire female rabbit lives in the garden with a run attached to her two-storey hutch (**17**). During the summer months it has been digging burrows to the extent that the owner's lawn has started to collapse. Although not ideal, the owner feels that there is no option but to move the rabbit and the run on to concrete to prevent the problem. Concerned that the rabbit was bored, the owner also purchased a male guinea pig as company. The owner would like to give both animals the chance to live on grass over the winter months. What advice would you give?

**CASE 18** On routine surgical exposure of the abdomen in rabbits, what anatomical structures are located immediately below the incision site and should therefore be carefully avoided (18)?

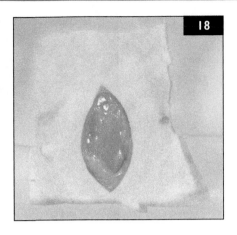

**CASE 19** An adult wild Eastern Cottontail rabbit is brought to a clinic in Texas, USA, in mid-July after being found near a private home. The man who found the rabbit said that it was acting strangely, rubbing its nose on the ground and twitching intermittently. The rabbit did not run away from him when he attempted to pick it up. On examination the rabbit is severely depressed, has a roughened hair coat and is reluctant to move. There are no skin lesions or bite wounds on the rabbit. The rabbit dies shortly after presentation.

1 Given the species and geographic location, what is your main differential diagnosis?
2 What is your next step?
3 How would you advise the man who brought the rabbit in?

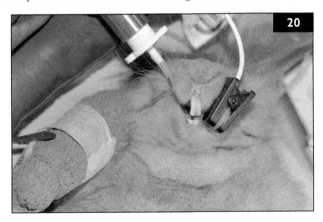

**CASE 20** What anaesthetic circuit and associated equipment is suitable for gaseous anaesthesia in rabbits (20)?

9

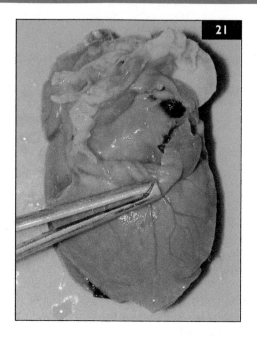

**CASE 21** An 8-year-old male neutered, crossbred house rabbit is acutely dyspnoeic. The animal collapses and dies suddenly on presentation.

1 What are the lesion(s) observed in the photograph (**21**) taken at postmortem examination?
2 What is the most likely cause of the postmortem changes in this animal?

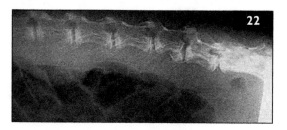

**CASE 22** A 1-year-old rabbit presents as an emergency with paralysed hindlimbs following a struggle by the owner to restrain it.

1 What lesion is shown in the lateral radiograph of the lumbar spine (**22**)?
2 How would you determine a prognosis, and what emergency treatment would you consider?

**CASE 23** An owner reports a fight between two rabbits that have been living together within the home for at least six months (**23**). The fight occurred within the doe's cage and has left the male rabbit with a severe injury to one eye. Each rabbit has its own indoor cage and the rabbits usually move happily from one cage to the other. Since the fight the rabbits have been separated and the owner is too scared to put them together again, although she is not happy with them living alone. What advice would you give about managing this situation?

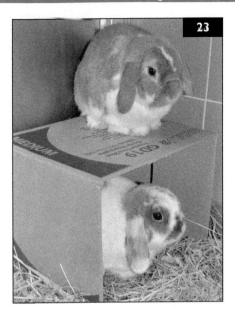

**CASE 24**
1 Name the vessels indicated in **24**.
2 Why should vessel **1** be used with care for blood sampling?

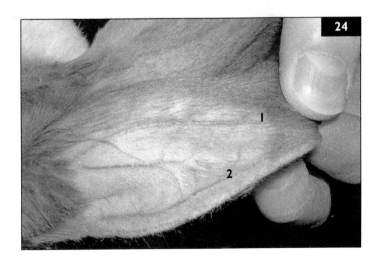

11

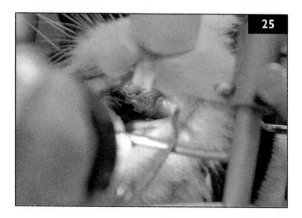

**CASE 25** A pet rabbit is inappetant following a lengthy dental procedure performed under sedation which identified and corrected dental spikes causing oral trauma (25).

1 Why is the rabbit likely to be inappetant?
2 What postoperative medication would be appropriate for this case?
3 What is the likely prognosis in this case?

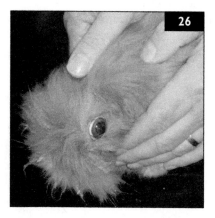

**CASE 26** A 6-year-old male neutered rabbit is presented with a history of gradual onset lethargy and bilateral exophthalmos (26). On physical examination both eyes can be retropulsed normally without obvious pain, but exophthalmos is worsened by ventroflexion.

1 What are your differential diagnoses?
2 What diagnostics would you recommend to confirm your diagnosis?

## CASE 27
1 What opioid analgesics are commonly used in rabbits, and what is their duration of action?
2 What can they be used for in addition to analgesia?
3 What are the undesirable side effects of opioids?

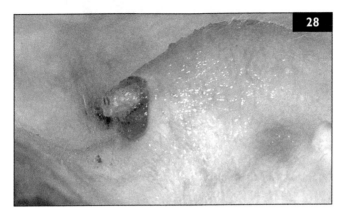

**CASE 28** A 2-year-old male castrated rabbit in the USA is housed in an outdoor hutch for the warm spring and summer months. The owner noticed an area of matted fur on the side of the rabbit's neck that seems painful. Otherwise, the rabbit seems bright and alert, is passing normal droppings and has a good appetite. The matted fur around the area is clipped and beneath it is found a subcutaneous swelling with a small hole at its tip (28).

1 What word best describes this condition?
2 Describe your treatment and prevention plan.

## CASE 29
1 What are the dental formulas (deciduous and permanent) of the rabbit (29)?
2 Describe the normal dental anatomy and function.

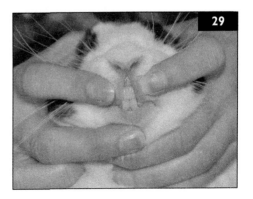

13

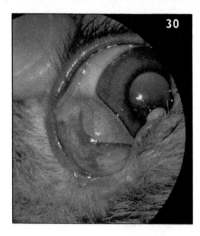

**CASE 30** A 3-year-old male neutered crossbred rabbit presents with a slowly progressive soft tissue mass at the medial canthus of the left eye. There is no apparent discomfort but the presence of the mass is leading to some tear overflow due to abnormal eyelid function.

1  What is the lesion (30)?
2  How would you treat this case?

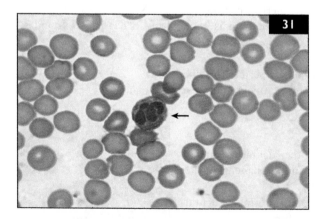

**CASE 31**
1  Identify the indicated cell on the rapid Romanovsky-type (Rapid-Diff) stained blood smear shown (31).
2  Is the morphology normal, and, if not, why?

**CASE 32** Two rabbits in the USA are housed in an outdoor hutch with an open wire mesh floor. A month prior to presentation the owner witnessed a raccoon trying to get into the hutch, and one of the rabbits sustained a bite wound to its hindlimb. The owner cleaned the wound with hydrogen peroxide and let it heal on its own. Now the owner reports this same rabbit is anorexic and trembling. On presentation, the rabbit is grinding its teeth, has a slight head tremor and is ataxic in the forelimbs. The other rabbit seems unaffected.

1 What is the most likely cause of this rabbit's clinical signs?
2 Should you do anything with the asymptomatic rabbit that also lives in the hutch?

**CASE 33** A small rabbit breeding facility has suffered a number of losses due to hepatic coccidiosis.

1 Hepatic coccidiosis increases the body's requirement for which two vitamins?
2 What clinical signs may be observed in rabbits with deficiencies of these two vitamins?

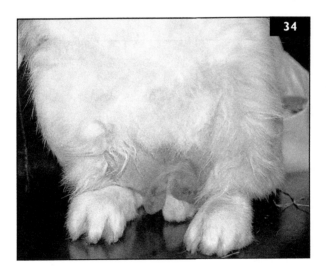

**CASE 34** A male rabbit 2 days post castration is shown (34).

1 What abnormalities can be seen?
2 What are the differential diagnoses, and what further investigative procedures should be carried out?

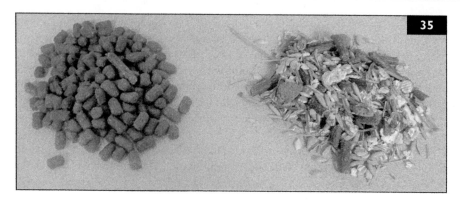

**CASE 35** Two types of commercially available concentrate foods are shown (35). The one on the left is an extruded pellet and the one on the right a mixed ration.

**1** Give one advantage and one disadvantage of each type of food over the other.
**2** Is either of these foods suitable as a complete *ad libitum* diet for adult or geriatric pet rabbits?
**3** How should these foods be stored?

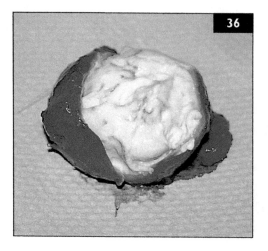

**CASE 36** An encapsulated abscess is shown, following its surgical removal from the subcutaneous tissue on the lateral neck (cervical region) of a rabbit (36). Describe how you would obtain a sample for bacterial culture in this case.

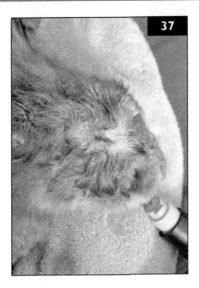

**CASE 37** What emergency procedures should you carry out in an anaesthetized rabbit in which respiratory arrest has occurred (37)?

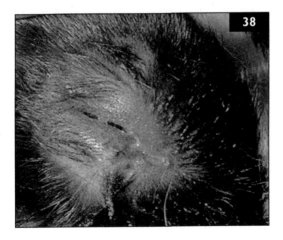

**CASE 38** A 2-year-old Dwarf Lop rabbit presents with acute swelling and discomfort of the right eye.

1  What is the condition shown (38)?
2  What diagnostic tests would you perform in this case, and how would you treat the patient while waiting for results?

17

**CASE 39** A 3-year-old female Netherland Dwarf rabbit underwent a general anaesthetic and dental procedure 7 days previously. The rabbit presents with acute onset severe inspiratory dyspnoea and open mouth breathing. The animal is very distressed, the mucous membranes are slightly cyanotic and the lung sounds are difficult to assess, with a pronounced respiratory stridor.

1 What immediate treatment would you consider?
2 What are the differential diagnoses for this rabbit?
3 How would you confirm your diagnosis?

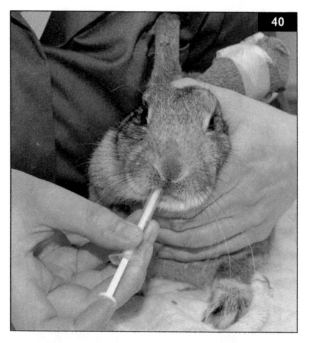

**CASE 40** What factors should be considered when deciding the route of administration of an antibiotic drug to a pet rabbit (40)?

## CASE 41
1 Give four examples of injectable balanced anaesthetic regimes suitable for surgical procedures.
2 Are any injectable anaesthetics licensed for use in the rabbit in the UK?

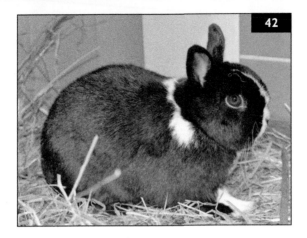

## CASE 42

1 If only 0.5 ml of blood is sampled from an 800 g Netherland Dwarf rabbit (42), which anticoagulant should be selected to allow both haematology and serum biochemistry to be performed on the same sample?
2 What is the disadvantage of selecting this anticoagulant for haematology?
3 Why is it inadvisable to flush the sampling syringe with heparin or heparin–saline before blood sampling?

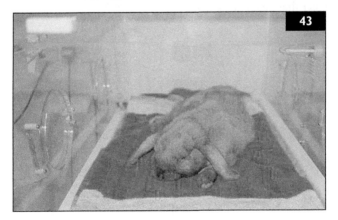

**CASE 43** This rabbit (43) is in an incubator, recovering from a surgical procedure.

1 What temperature should the incubator be set at initially and as the rabbit recovers further?
2 List the other components of supportive care that the rabbit should receive in the postoperative period.

19

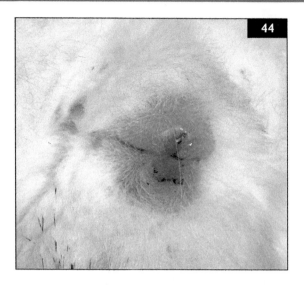

**CASE 44** A pet rabbit is presented with oedematous swelling of the anogenital area (44).

1 What are your differential diagnoses?
2 What further diagnostic tests would you perform?

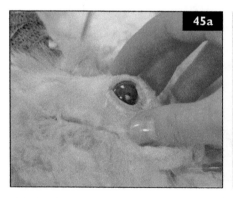
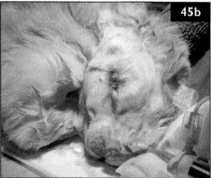

**CASE 45** Describe how you would perform an enucleation in a rabbit (45a, b). How does this surgical procedure differ in the rabbit compared with enucleation in cats and dogs?

## CASE 46

1 What are the indications for the use of an antimuscarinic (parasympatholytic) agent in rabbit anaesthetic protocols?
2 What agent is most suitable in this species and why?
3 What commonly used drug in rabbits can be antagonized by antimuscarinics?

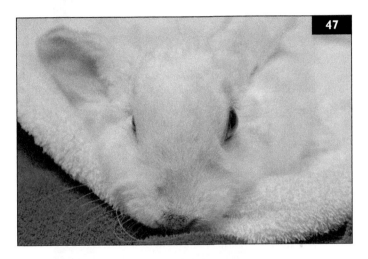

**CASE 47** A 1-year-old pet rabbit presents with unilateral exophthalmos and a history of anorexia and excessive salivation (**47**).

1 What are the differential diagnoses in this case?
2 What further investigative procedures would you perform?

## CASE 48

1 What cestode infections occur in rabbits, and how do they present?
2 What is the treatment of choice for cestode infection in rabbits?

**CASE 49** Explain the terms diphyodont, heterodont and aradicular hypsodont, which describe the dental anatomy and physiology of the rabbit, and comment on the clinical significance of aradicular hypsodont.

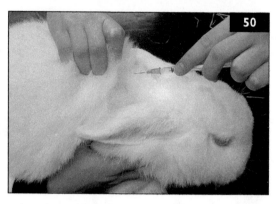

**CASE 50** Ketamine, butorphanol and medetomidine may be given as a pre-euthanasia anaesthetic combination. A small volume of the combined drugs is injected subcutaneously (s/c) (50).

1 What are the advantages of inducing anaesthesia prior to euthanasia in a pet rabbit?
2 What are the advantages of using this particular anaesthetic combination?
3 What are the disadvantages of using this particular anaesthetic combination?

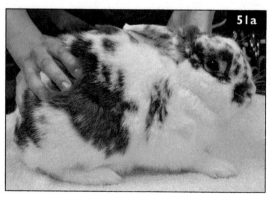

**CASE 51** An outdoor rabbit presents with a soft-tissue swelling on the shoulder (51a). On palpation, the structure feels fluid filled and you suspect a cyst. You aspirate fluid and confirm microscopically the presence of tapeworm scolices.

1 What is the most likely species of tapeworm causing this problem?
2 What is the tapeworm lifecycle?
3 What treatment plan do you advise?
4 How can you prevent rabbits from developing this infection?

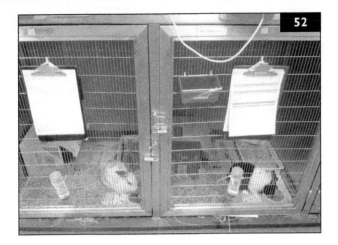

**CASE 52** What essential physical assessments and daily observations of a hospitalized rabbit (52) are required, at least at the beginning of the day, to enable an informed patient assessment?

**CASE 53** Comment on the use of nitrous oxide in rabbit anaesthesia.

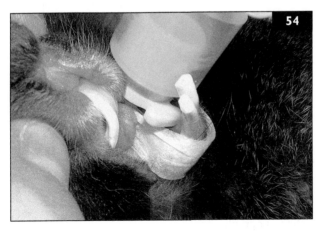

**CASE 54** The mouth of an anaesthetized and intubated 4-month-old rabbit with an obvious dental abnormality is shown (54).

1  What is the condition shown, and what is the most likely aetiology in this case?
2  What treatment/management options are available?

23

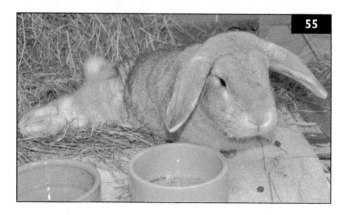

**CASE 55** A 2-year-old rabbit presents with acute onset posterior paresis (55). What are the differential diagnoses?

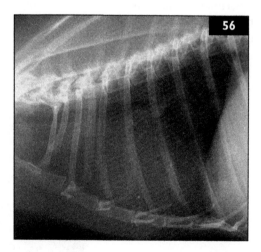

**CASE 56** A 3-year-old Netherland Dwarf rabbit presents with mild lethargy and decreased appetite. On thoracic auscultation the lung sounds are moderately increased, with some crackles heard. A lateral thoracic radiograph is taken (56).

1  What does the radiograph reveal?
2  What are your differential diagnoses?


**CASE 57** Describe how you would auscultate the thorax of a rabbit.

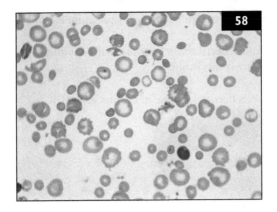

**CASE 58** A rapid Romanovsky-type (Rapid-Diff) stained blood smear from a 7-year-old neutered female Dwarf Lop house rabbit, with a severe regenerative anaemia, is shown (**58**). The PCV was 0.14 l/l (14%); Hb was 27 g/l (2.7 g/dl). The rabbit was presented with gradually increasing lethargy and decreased appetite of several weeks' duration.

1 Characterize the anaemia from the red cell morphology.
2 What stain may be used to differentiate reticulocytes more accurately?
3 What is the most likely cause of this anaemia, and give a differential diagnosis.
4 What other haematological and biochemistry abnormalities may occur with this condition?

**CASE 59**

1 What technique is being used in this rabbit (**59**)?
2 How is it performed, and what are its applications?

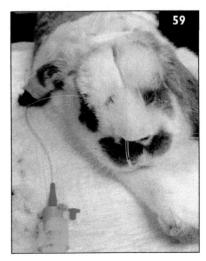

**CASE 60** The rabbit in case 56 has bronchopneumonia.

1  What are the major contributing factors to this condition?
2  How would you treat this rabbit?

**CASE 61** Buserelin is licensed for use in rabbits in the UK. What is it indicated for and what is its mode of action?

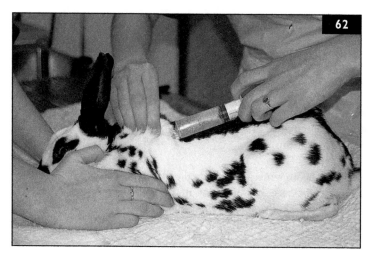

**CASE 62** What is the maximum volume per kg body weight that should be administered by s/c injection in rabbits (62)?

**CASE 63**
1  Describe how you determine the sex of a rabbit.
2  When is the best age to sex rabbit kits?
3  At what age do rabbits become sexually mature?

**CASE 64** A 2-year-old pet rabbit with diarrhoea is to be hospitalized for fluid therapy. What are the basic housing requirements for hospitalized rabbits?

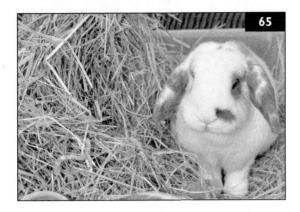

CASE 65 Meadow and grass hays (65) are a very good source of dietary fibre and should make up the bulk of rabbit diets.

1 In relation to rabbit digestive physiology, what do the terms digestible fibre and indigestible fibre refer to?
2 Discuss the health benefits of a diet high in indigestible fibre.
3 Other than hay, what foods provide a source of fibre?

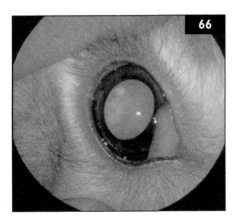

CASE 66 A 2-year-old rabbit presents with a recent history of progressive loss of vision associated with bilateral cataracts (66). What are the causes of cataract formation in the rabbit, and what advice would you give the owner on the possibility of restoring sight?

27

CASE 67 A 1-year-old female rabbit has blood taken before a routine ovariohysterectomy is performed. The results are shown in the table.

| | SI units | Range |
|---|---|---|
| RBCs | $6.16 \times 10^{12}$/l | (4.8–7.2) |
| Hb | 126 g/l | (103–155) |
| PCV | 0.41 l/l | (0.35–0.48) |
| MCV | 64.7 fl | (61–76) |
| MCHC | 320 g/l | (282–342) |
| WBCs | $4.6 \times 10^9$/l | (3.3–12.0) |
| AST | 54 iu/l | (6.7–54.2) |
| ALT | 29 iu/l | (22.1–80.2) |
| GGT | 6 iu/l | (0–7.0) |
| LDH | 857 iu/l | (<1500) |
| TP | 64 g/l | (53–79) |
| Albumin | 40 g/l | (35.9–41.4) |
| Globulin | 24 g/l | (11.6–43.1) |
| Urea | 6.8 mmol/l | (3.0–9.5) |
| Creatinine | 87 μmol/l | (71–256) |
| Calcium | 4.34 mmol/l | (1.9–3.6) |
| CK/CPK | 322 iu/l | (140–372) |
| Triglyceride | 2.7 mmol/l | (2.6–3.5) |

What is the significance of the elevated value, and what is the likely cause?

## CASE 68

1 Describe the oestrous cycle of the rabbit.
2 How should a buck and doe be introduced for mating?
3 What is the gestation period and what methods of pregnancy diagnosis are possible in the rabbit?

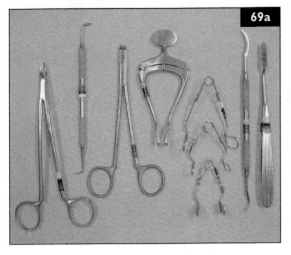
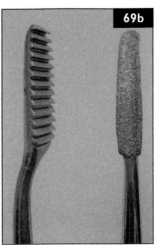

**CASE 69** An assortment of tools commonly used for rabbit dentistry is shown (69a, b).

1 Identify the tools and describe their uses.
2 Which of the tools in **69b** would you choose for inclusion in your dental kit? Explain your preference.

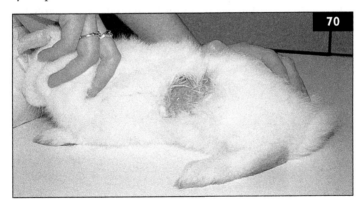

**CASE 70** An owner reports that her rabbit's skin is very loose and extensible and that it tore when she was grooming it (70).

1 What underlying condition would you suspect?
2 How would you confirm your diagnosis?
3 How would you treat this rabbit?

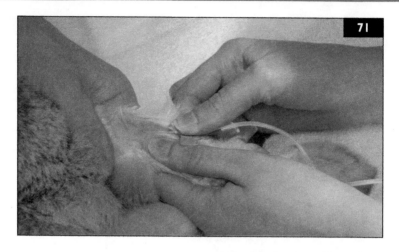

**CASE 71** What volume of blood can be safely collected at any one time in a 2 kg pet rabbit (71), and how is this calculated?

**CASE 72** A rabbit presents with a bilateral nasal discharge of 3-week duration but is clinically bright with a good appetite.

1 What are your differential diagnoses for bilateral nasal discharge in a rabbit?
2 What diagnostic tests could you perform?

**CASE 73** A 5-year-old male neutered Angora rabbit with a history of chronic upper respiratory disease due to a mixed bacterial infection insidiously develops a head tilt to the right-hand side and generalized ataxia over a 2-month period. On examination, there is a slow bilateral rotatory nystagmus. A blood sample is taken for *Encephalitozoon cuniculi* serology and proves to be negative. A series

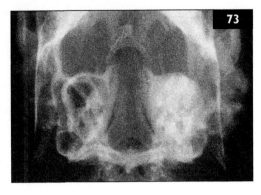

of skull radiographs is taken and the images consistently reveal an increase in the radiopacity of one of the tympanic bullae (73).

1 What could this increase in radiopacity represent?
2 What diagnostic modality would provide further detail to assess the bullae?
3 What is the most likely diagnosis?
4 In the event that medical treatment is ineffective, are there any surgical options for treatment of such a case?
5 What postoperative complications could be expected with this technique?

**CASE 74** A 5-year-old British Giant rabbit lives outside in a hutch and run (74). For the past 6 months the rabbit has been thumping her back feet for several hours from approximately 2 a.m. onwards. The owner has had complaints from the neighbours as the sound is waking them. The owner is adamant that there are no foxes around, as she has looked out of the window when the behaviour has just started. What advice would you give to

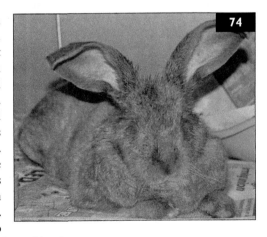

this owner on how to deal with this problem?

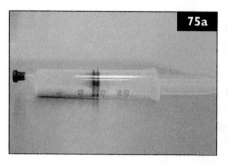

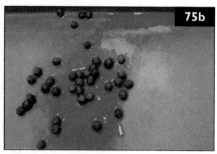

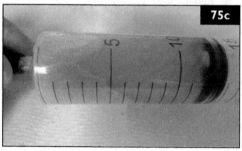

**CASE 75** A urine sample from an apparently healthy adult female French Lop rabbit is shown (**75a, b, c**). Semi-quantitative urinalysis using a urine test strip gives the following results: pH – 8; protein – +; glucose – negative; ketones – negative. All other urine dipstick parameters are negative. The SG, measured with a refractometer, is 1.028.

1  What is the likely cause of the urine colour?
2  What is the likely cause of the turbidity?

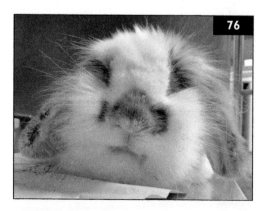

**CASE 76** *Pasteurella multocida* is commonly involved in respiratory disease in rabbits (**76**). How can this infection be controlled and prevented?

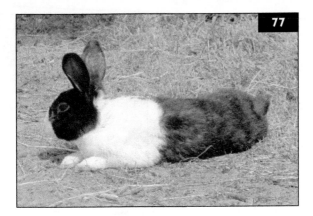

**CASE 77** A 10-year-old male entire rabbit is presented due to reduced activity levels and problems grooming its back end (**77**).

1 What would your approach be to this case?
2 What supportive treatment would you recommend?

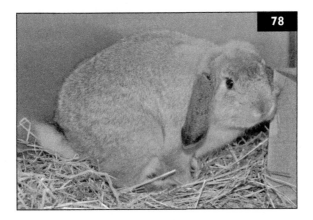

**CASE 78** A female rabbit neutered 8 months ago has recently started to build a nest (**78**). She has also changed from being a gentle and friendly rabbit to grunting at the owner and being unwilling to be stroked. The owner cannot report any husbandry changes that may be relevant to this problem. What advice would you give to the client?

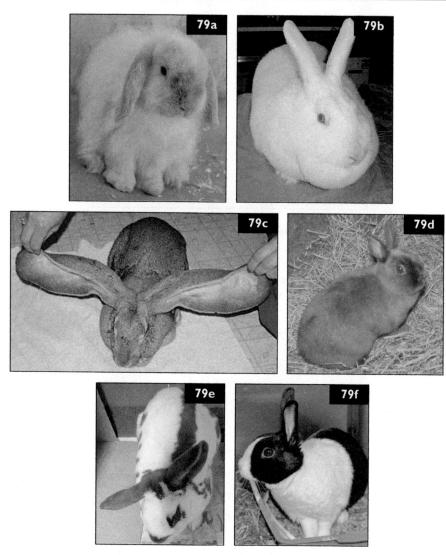

**CASE 79** Identify these rabbit breeds (79a–f).

**CASE 80** What are the common venepuncture sites in the rabbit, and what are their relative advantages/disadvantages?

**CASE 81** A 1-year-old rabbit presents with a history of recent appearance of a white opacity in the left eye (81). There is no discomfort.

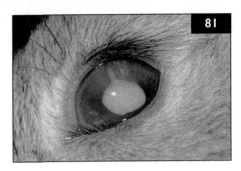

1 What is the most likely diagnosis in this case, and what are the possible aetiologies?
2 How would you investigate and treat this condition?

## CASE 82
1 Describe the dentistry applications for the instruments shown (82a, b, c).
2 What precautions are required for their safe use in each case?

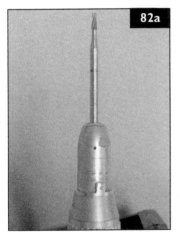

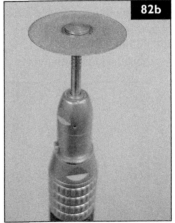

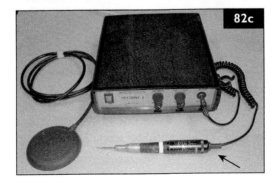

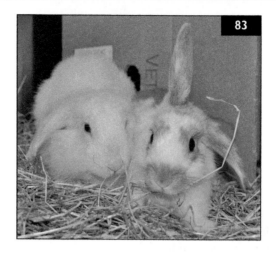

## CASE 83

1 What advice would you give a client keen to keep pet rabbits as to the ideal number and sex combination (83)?
2 How should unfamiliar rabbits be introduced to each other?
3 Should rabbits be kept with guinea pigs?

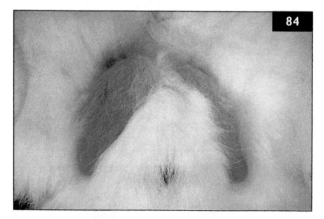

**CASE 84** Why is castration recommended in male rabbits (84), and what is the recommended age for this procedure?

**CASE 85** Describe how you would collect blood from the marginal ear vein of a pet rabbit.

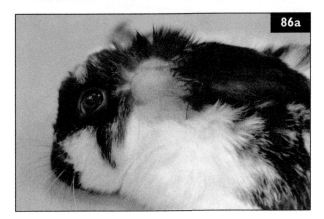

**CASE 86** An owner brings his Lop rabbit in for a routine vaccination. As part of your physical examination you notice bilateral painful soft tissue swellings at the base of the ears (**86a**).

1  What is the likely diagnosis?
2  How would you confirm your diagnosis?
3  What treatment options could be offered to the owner?

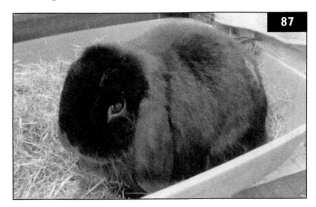

**CASE 87** An 8-year-old female neutered rabbit is presented for an annual health check (**87**). Another of the owner's rabbits has recently been euthanased due to renal failure and the owner asks for advice about potential problems in the older rabbit.

1  What is the lifespan for a pet rabbit?
2  What common problems are seen in geriatric rabbits?
3  What preventive healthcare advice would you give for the geriatric rabbit?

37

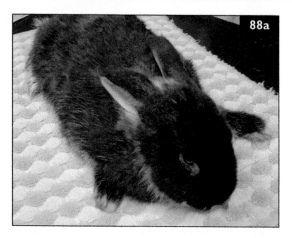

88a

**CASE 88** A 1-year-old pet rabbit presents in a collapsed and hypovolaemic state (**88a**).

1  Describe how you would administer fluid therapy to this animal.
2  What type of fluids would you use and at what flow rate?

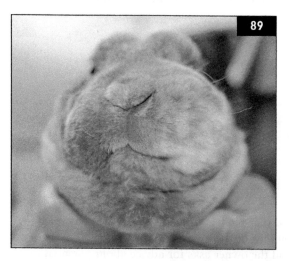

89

**CASE 89** A rabbit presents with a subcutaneous swelling on its face (**89**). List your differential diagnoses for subcutaneous facial swellings in rabbits.

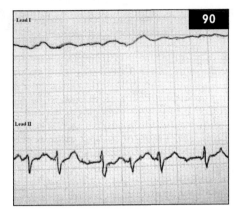

**CASE 90** A 6-year-old New Zealand White rabbit presented collapsed, in thin body condition and with moderate dyspnoea. Pulse deficits and an irregular heart rhythm with tachycardia (280 bpm) were detected on clinical examination. An electrocardiogram was taken at the time (**90**).

1 What is your diagnosis?
2 How would you treat this condition?

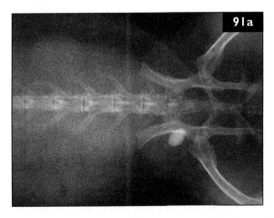

**CASE 91** A 3-year-old male neutered rabbit presents with signs of dysuria, perineal urine staining, lethargy and anorexia. On clinical examination, palpation of the caudal abdomen is resented. A ventrodorsal abdominal radiograph is taken (**91a**).

1 What is seen in the radiograph?
2 Describe the surgical management of this case.
3 What postoperative care is indicated?

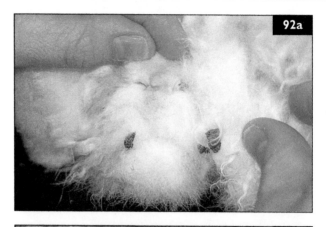

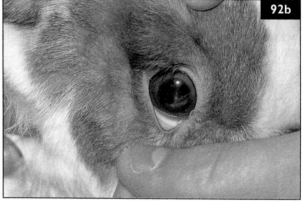

**CASE 92** A 3-year-old Dwarf Lop house rabbit presents with anorexia and lethargy. The owner has noticed the rabbit stripping paint off the wall in a corner of one room. On clinical examination there is pallor of the mucous membranes (92a, b).

1 What further diagnostic tests would you perform?
2 What is your likely diagnosis, and how would you confirm this?
3 What treatment is indicated?

**CASE 93** List the measures that can be taken in a veterinary practice to minimize the stress experienced by the rabbit patient.

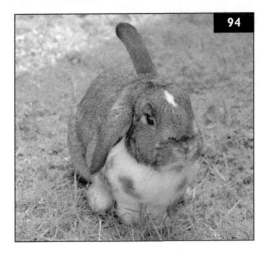

**CASE 94** This rabbit is outside on a hot sunny day (**94**).

1  How do rabbits thermoregulate?
2  How do they cope with extremes of cold and heat?

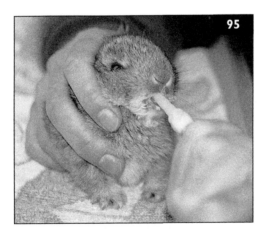

**CASE 95** This rabbit kit is being hand reared (**95**).

1  What situations can lead to this procedure being necessary, and how can you assess if kits require hand rearing?
2  What are the common causes of failure of hand reared kits to thrive or survive?
3  What housing and temperature is appropriate for hand rearing?

**CASE 96** What are the intramuscular injection sites in rabbits?

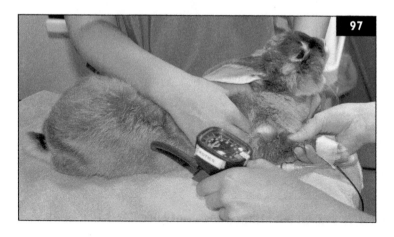

**CASE 97**

1 What procedure is being carried out (97)?
2 What is the most likely reason for carrying out this procedure in a pet rabbit?

**CASE 98** An adult male house rabbit is admitted to hospital with a history of 3 days' anorexia. This is due to molar spurs, which have lacerated the tongue and are visible on oral examination with an otoscope. The rabbit is anaesthetized and the spurs burred. The rabbit is kept hospitalized, and it is given meloxicam analgesia, metoclopramide and ranitidine to help prevent ileus, as well being syringe fed a high-fibre gruel. After 3 days the rabbit is producing some normal faecal pellets but remains anorexic. A urine sample is collected from the floor of the hospital cage. The urine is tested with a urine dipstick, the SG measured with a refractometer, and the urine sediment examined. These are the findings: SG = 1.026; pH = 6.0; protein = +; glucose = +; ketones = +++. All other dipstick parameters are negative.

1 Which parameters are normal and which are abnormal?
2 What is the significance of these findings, and what is the likely reason for the rabbit's continued anorexia?

**CASE 99** What type of treatment is being carried out (99)?

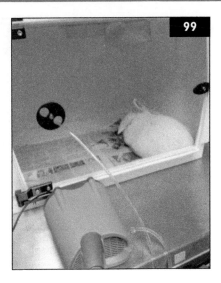

**CASE 100** A 2-year-old male Dutch rabbit has been obtained directly from the breeder at 20 months old. The owner has bought the rabbit a large two-tiered hutch and is trying to spend an hour a day with him. He is a very nervous rabbit and will avoid his owner if she tries to pick him up. The owner reports aggression if she does not leave him alone when he is 'worked up'. She would like to have him castrated in the hope that he will calm down. What advice would you give this owner?

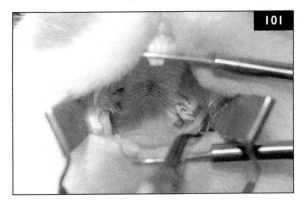

**CASE 101** Acquired dental disease is a common problem in pet rabbits that is not generally seen in wild rabbits (101).

1  Outline the aetiology of acquired dental disease.
2  Describe the progression of dental changes.

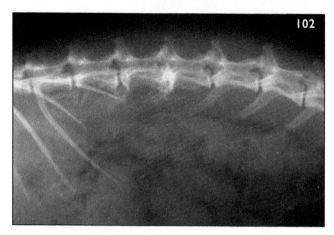

**CASE 102** A lateral radiograph of the lumbar spine of a 7-year-old rabbit is shown (**102**).

1 What condition is illustrated?
2 What clinical signs may be associated with this condition, and how can the condition be treated?

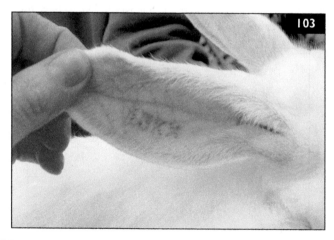

**CASE 103** This rabbit has been identified by a tattoo in its ear (**103**).

1 What other methods of individually identifying rabbits are used?
2 What method is required for exhibition purposes in the UK?

## CASE 104

1 What procedure is being shown (104)?
2 What anatomical sites may be used for this procedure?
3 Describe the technique.

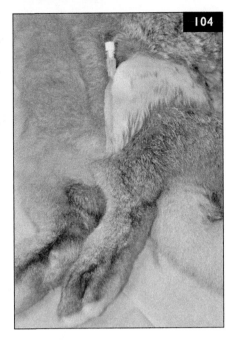

CASE 105 External skeletal fixation is a useful technique for the repair of many fractures seen in rabbits (105).

1 What are the advantages and disadvantages of using this method of fixation?
2 What factor influences the decision to use an open versus a closed surgical approach for placement of the fixator pins?
3 What speed and angle are suitable for the placement of the pins?

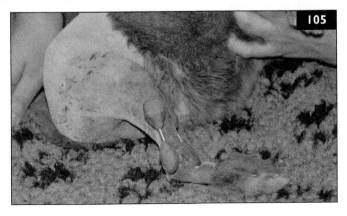

## CASE 106

1 What is the expected lifespan of a pet rabbit?
2 What factors will affect lifespan?
3 Is it possible to age a rabbit?

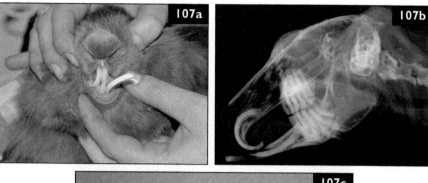

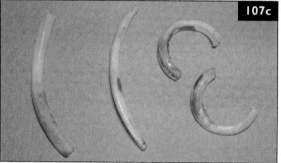

**CASE 107** Incisor malocclusion is not uncommon in rabbits (**107a, b**). The incisors extracted from a rabbit with congenital incisor malocclusion are shown (**107c**) (peg teeth not shown).

1 Which are the upper and which are the lower incisors?
2 Describe the extraction technique and postoperative care required.
3 What additional considerations are there in cases of acquired incisor malocclusion?

## CASE 108

1 Give the order, family, subfamily, genus and species of the domestic rabbit.
2 How many chromosomes does the domestic rabbit possess?
3 To what genus do wild American rabbits belong?
4 Are Jack rabbits true rabbits?
5 Are Belgian hares true hares?

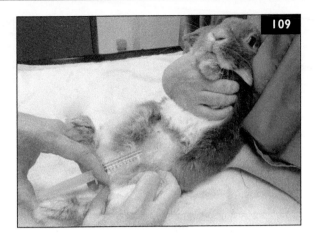

## CASE 109
1 What injection technique is being shown (109)?
2 What are the potential complications associated with this procedure in the rabbit?

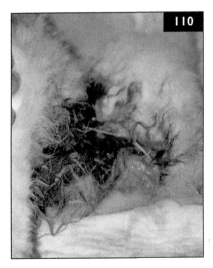

**CASE 110** This rabbit presents to you with soft faecal material adhered to the fur around its perineum (110). The owner reports that it has diarrhoea.

1 How can you determine if this is indeed true diarrhoea?
2 If you determine that true diarrhoea is not present, what can cause this presentation?

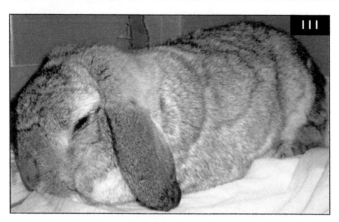

**CASE 111** An adult, neutered male domestic rabbit is presented with lethargy, depression and anorexia of a few days' duration (**111**). On physical examination the rabbit appears in fairly good body condition. A blood sample is collected and urinalysis performed. The findings revealed azotemia and concurrent hyposthenuria. What is your diagnosis, and how would you manage this case?

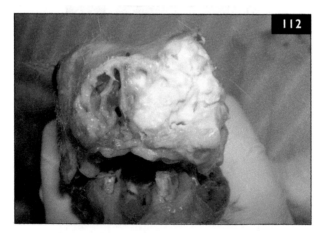

**CASE 112** An adult, female rabbit from a private breeder was euthanased after a chronic history of sneezing and nasal secretion, non-responsive to antibiotics. The postmortem frontal section of the nasal cavity of this rabbit (**112**) shows accumulation of semisolid purulent material with associated bone destruction of the left nasal cavity.

1 What is the most common leukocyte found in rabbit pus?
2 What is the bacterium most commonly isolated from rabbit pus?

**CASE 113** An 8-week-old female Dutch rabbit, bought from a pet shop 3 days previously, presents severely depressed, with anorexia and a small amount of very soft green-brown faeces soiling the fur of the perineum. The rabbit is admitted to the hospital and a jugular blood sample taken. These are the results:

|  | SI units | Range |
|---|---|---|
| RBC | $7.6 \times 10^{12}/l$* | (4.8–7.2) |
| Hb | 152 g/l | (103–155) |
| PCV | 0.51 l/l* | (0.35–0.48) |
| WBCs | $9.8 \times 10^9/l$ | (3.3–12.0) |
| Neutrophils | $9.02 \times 10^9/l$* | (2.6–6.0) |
| Lymphocytes | $0.59 \times 10^9/l$* | (1.8–6.3) |
| Monocytes | $0.19 \times 10^9/l$ | (0–1.8) |
| AST | 62 iu/l* | (6.7–54.2) |
| ALT | 118 iu/l* | (22.1–80.2) |
| ALP | 146 iu/l* | (15.1–19.3) |
| GGT | 5 iu/l | (0–7.0) |
| LDH | 1184 iu/l | (<1500) |
| TP | 87 g/l* | (53–79) |
| Albumin | 45 g/l* | (35.9–41.4) |
| Globulin | 42 g/l | (11.6–43.1) |
| Urea | 7.8 mmol/l | (3.0–9.5) |
| Creatinine | 223 μmol/l | (71–256) |
| Calcium | 3.1 mmol/l | (1.9–3.6) |
| CK/CPK | 327 iu/l | (140–372) |
| Triglyceride | 2.9 mmol/l | (2.6–3.5) |
| Glucose | 14.8 mmol/l* | (4.2–8.3) |

1 What do the abnormalities marked with an asterisk indicate?
2 What is the likely diagnosis?

49

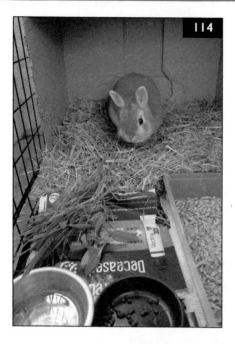

## CASE 114

1 What levels of dietary fibre, fat and protein are appropriate for adult pet rabbits (**114**)?

2 How do the nutritional requirements of lactating does and growing juveniles differ from those of non-breeding adults?

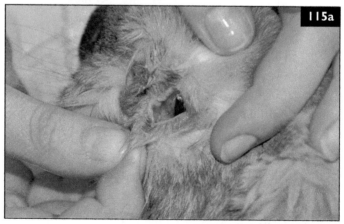

**CASE 115** This rabbit (**115a**) is displaying what is often the earliest sign of acquired dental disease.

1 What is the condition, and how is it related to the teeth?

2 What other indicators of dental disease might be apparent on routine physical examination, even before inspecting the oral cavity?

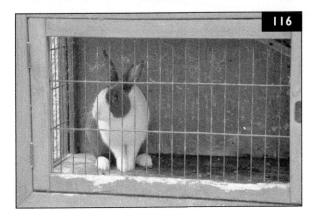

**CASE 116** This rabbit is kept permanently in an outdoor hutch (**116**).

1 Is this suitable accommodation?
2 What advice would you give an owner on the minimum size of a hutch?

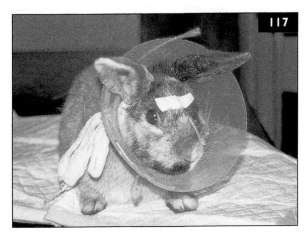

**CASE 117** Describe the method of placement of a nasogastric tube in a rabbit (**117**). What are the potential complications associated with this technique?

**CASE 118** What are the commonly observed post-castration complications in rabbits, and how may these be avoided?

51

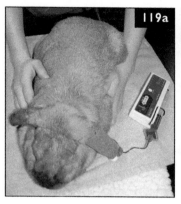 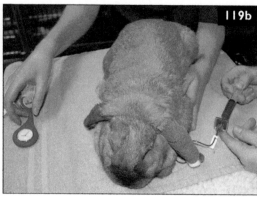

## CASE 119
1 What is the procedure being performed (119a, b)?
2 For what conditions is this procedure indicated?

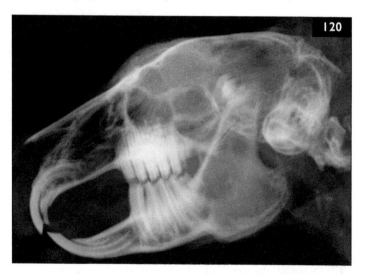

CASE 120 What are the standard radiographic views used for imaging in the rabbit (120)?

CASE 121 What plants are known to cause toxicity in rabbits?

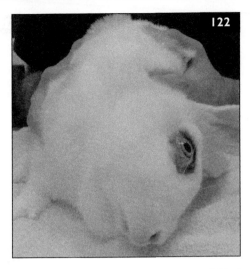

**CASE 122** A 3-year-old neutered female domestic rabbit is presented with a sudden onset left-sided head tilt (**122**). Encephalitozoonosis infection is a primary differential diagnosis. What auxiliary test could be used for the *in vivo* diagnosis of active Encephalitozoonosis in this case, alongside measurement of antibody titres?

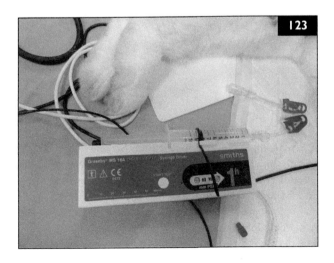

**CASE 123** This rabbit has just undergone a partial ear canal ablation and bulla osteotomy. It is currently receiving i/v fluids via an intravenous syringe driver (**123**). How would you optimize analgesia during the immediate postoperative period and ensure that an adequate level of analgesia is maintained throughout?

53

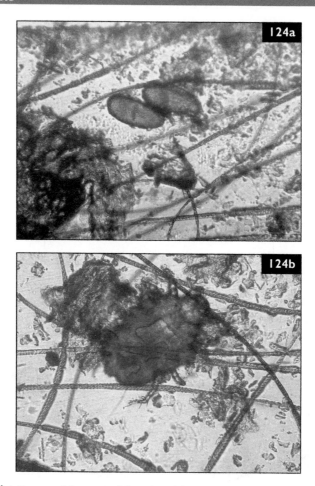

**CASE 124** A 2-year-old neutered female rabbit presents with some skin scale and mild alopecia over the dorsal interscapular region. The owner is unsure whether the rabbit is pruritic or not. A cellotape impression is examined by microscopy. Eggs are found attached to the hairs, and a single mite is found (**124a, b**).

1 Identify the indicated mite and eggs.
2 What are the identifying features?
3 Which related organism is not generally associated with seborrhoea?

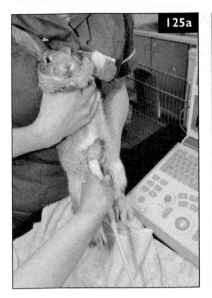
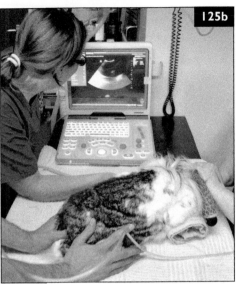

**CASE 125** What common conditions can be diagnosed on ultrasonographic examination of the urogenital tract in the female rabbit (125a, b)?

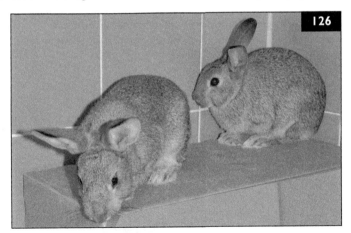

**CASE 126** Young rabbits (126) are frequently sold at 7 or 8 weeks of age having had minimal human contact. This is very different to the situation with pet kittens and puppies.

1  What problems can be caused in rabbits by lack of early socialization?
2  How can these problems be prevented?

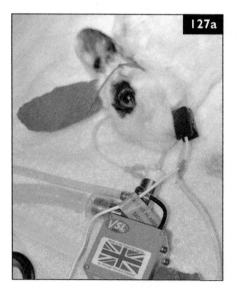

**CASE 127** What preoperative and intraoperative considerations are essential in rabbits undergoing a surgical procedure (127a)?

**CASE 128** Vitamin D acts as both a vitamin and a hormone in the body and has a range of physiological effects.

1 What potential sources of vitamin D are available to rabbits?
2 A reduced intestinal absorption of which mineral is likely to result from a chronic vitamin D deficiency in rabbits?
3 How might vitamin D toxicity present?

**CASE 129** A lateral abdominal radiograph from a rabbit is shown (129). What normal anatomical features can be seen?

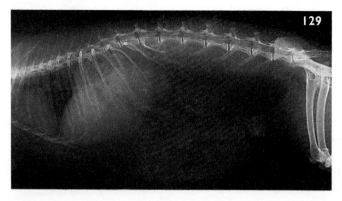

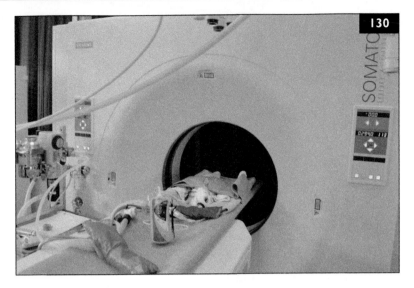

## CASE 130

1  What procedure is being carried out (130)?
2  For what conditions is this indicated in the rabbit?

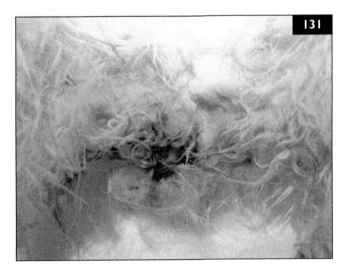

**CASE 131** A litter of 7-week-old rabbits from a breeder presents with profuse watery diarrhoea (131), dehydration, depression and anorexia. One of the litter has died. List the differential diagnoses for infectious causes of diarrhoea in rabbits of this age.

57

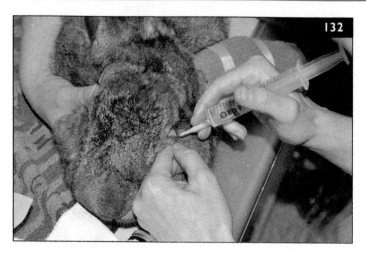

## CASE 132

1  What procedure is depicted (132)?
2  In what circumstances is this procedure indicated?

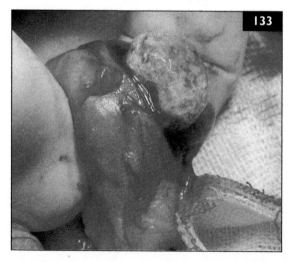

CASE 133 This intra-operative photograph shows a nephrotomy being performed in an adult domestic rabbit (133).

1  What is your diagnosis based on this photograph?
2  What are the most likely causes of this condition in pet rabbits?
3  How would you manage this case?

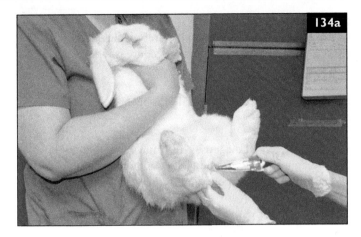

**CASE 134** It is important to assess the body temperature in a rabbit recovering from an anaesthetic.

1 What is the normal rectal temperature range in a rabbit (**134a**)?
2 At what body temperature in a rabbit would you start to be concerned about the risk of hypothermia?
3 What strategies would you employ to maintain normothermia?

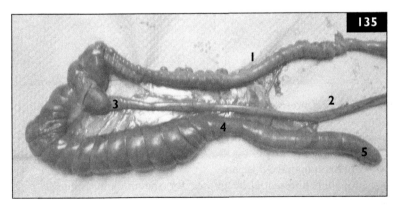

**CASE 135** A section of the GI tract of a young rabbit is shown (**135**).

1 Name the structures **1, 2, 3, 4** and **5**.
2 Describe the movement of ingesta through these portions of the GI system.

### CASE 136

1 Describe the procedure for collection of cerebrospinal fluid in the rabbit.
2 What are the conditions in which this procedure is indicated?

### CASE 137

A 5-year-old neutered female rabbit presents with urine scalding of the perineal area.

1 What are your differential diagnoses for urine scalding in rabbits?
2 What initial diagnostic tests would be advisable to perform?
3 Describe two ways you could obtain a sterile urine sample from this animal.

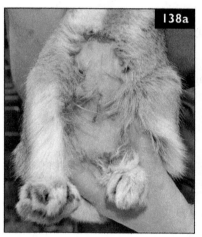 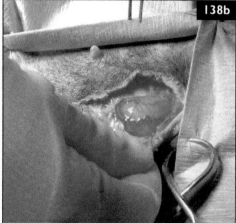

### CASE 138

A doe presents 4 days post ovariohysterectomy with anorexia and a swelling at the caudal edge of her midline abdominal incision (**138a**). Under general anaesthetic, you reopen the incision to see this sight (**138b**).

1 How would you manage this case?
2 What are your differential diagnoses for the midline swellings post spay procedure?
3 How would you determine if a case requires corrective surgery?

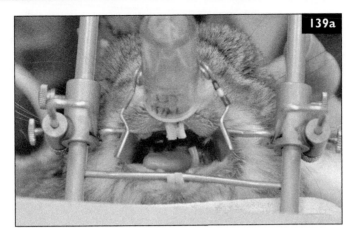

CASE 139 The photograph was taken during the dental treatment of a rabbit with acquired dental disease, and it shows an abnormal overgrowth of the lower left 1st premolar (139a).

1 What are the objectives of any rabbit dental treatment?
2 What technique can be used for dental correction?
3 Do dental rasps have a place in rabbit dental procedures?
4 What is the likely prognosis for this rabbit?

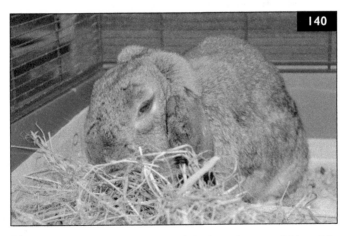

CASE 140 A collapsed and severely dehydrated pet rabbit with advanced myxomatosis is brought to the surgery (140). Euthanasia is advised on welfare grounds. It is not possible to find a suitable vein for i/v administration of barbiturate. What alternative methods of euthanasia could be used?

61

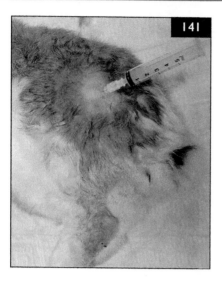

**CASE 141**
1 What procedure is being carried out on this cadaver (141)?
2 Describe how this is performed on a live rabbit.
3 For what conditions is this procedure indicated?

**CASE 142** Epizootic rabbit enteropathy (ERE) is a serious condition that first appeared in breeding colonies in the west of France in 1996 and has since been reported in a number of other European countries.

1 What age group does this disease primarily affect?
2 What are the associated clinical signs?
3 How is the disease diagnosed?
4 Which antimicrobial drugs have been shown to be of some benefit in reducing mortality rates or preventing outbreaks of the disease?

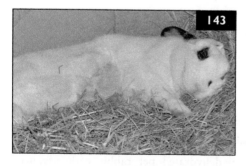

**CASE 143** A 4-year-old female rabbit presents with a history of anorexia of 24-hour duration and acute onset seizure activity (143). The owner reports two seizures in the last 24 hours, each consisting of paddling of all four limbs and lasting approximately 3 minutes.

1 What are your differential diagnoses?
2 What further diagnostic tests would you perform?
3 What are the treatment options?

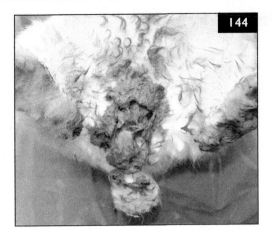

CASE 144 A colleague has been treating a 2-year-old rabbit with a respiratory tract infection with a long-acting s/c injection of amoxicillin-clavulanate. Two days later the rabbit has developed acute diarrhoea and is presented in a collapsed state (144).

1 What is the most likely diagnosis?
2 What is the prognosis?
3 What are the treatment options?

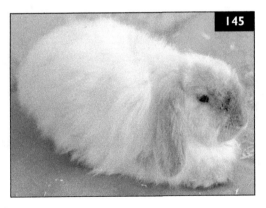

CASE 145 An indoor rabbit has been seen eating the leaves of one of the owner's houseplants (145). The owner is concerned that this may be toxic to the rabbit, although no adverse clinical signs have been noted. What is your advice?

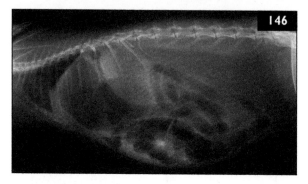

**CASE 146** A 2-year-old neutered female presents with a 1-day history of anorexia and mild depression. Clinical examination is unremarkable except for a slightly distended abdomen and lack of borborygmi. A lateral abdominal radiograph is taken (**146**).

1 What condition is seen in this radiograph?
2 What factors can affect gut motility?
3 What treatment would you initiate?

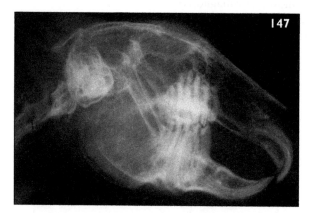

**CASE 147** Skull radiography or CT are essential for a complete assessment of the dentition. A lateral radiograph of a rabbit with advanced acquired dental disease is shown (**147**).

1 What information, relevant to the dentition, can be gained from radiography?
2 What standard views should be obtained?
3 Describe the radiographic features of acquired dental disease, with reference to any abnormalities in the picture.

**CASE 148** An owner asks about deworming her pet rabbit. What is your advice?

**CASE 149** A complication commonly seen in debilitated rabbit patients is hypothermia.

1 What is the normal rectal temperature of a rabbit?
2 What methods can be used to warm a hypothermic rabbit patient, and how is this achieved?

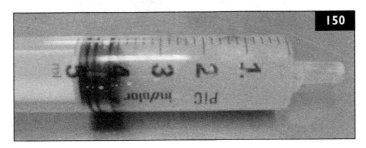

**CASE 150** A domestic rabbit is presented with weight loss and polydipsia, and you are suspicious of renal disease. How would you collect a urine sample (150), and what simple adjunct test could be performed on this sample to evaluate renal function?

**CASE 151** A 3-year-old male rabbit is presented with anorexia, depression, excess salivation and hindlimb weakness (151). The rabbit has spent the day grazing on the lawn of the owner, who had not realized that the gardener had recently treated the area with a fungicide.

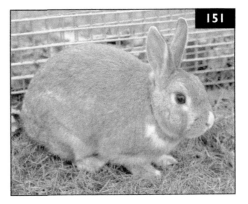

1 What toxin is likely to be involved?
2 What treatment is indicated?
3 What is the prognosis?

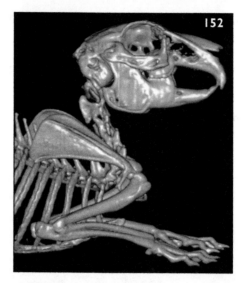

**CASE 152** The photograph shows part of a rabbit skeleton (**152**).

**1** What skeletal injuries are rabbits prone to if they are handled incorrectly?
**2** List the factors that make them susceptible to these injuries.

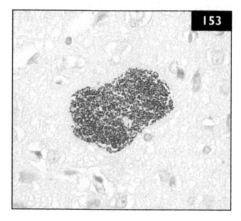

**CASE 153** A Gram-stained histological section from a rabbit's cerebrum is shown (**153**). The animal presented with severe head tilt and collapse. It was euthanased on welfare grounds.

**1** What is your diagnosis?
**2** How is this disease transmitted?

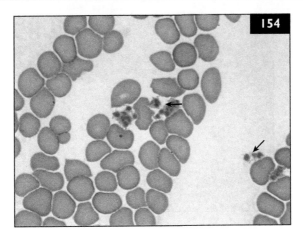

**CASE 154** What are the indicated structures on the rapid Romanovsky-type (Rapid-Diff) stained blood smear from a 3-year-old female French Lop rabbit (154)?

**CASE 155** A 2-year-old female neutered rabbit presents with sudden onset circling and a right-sided head tilt (155a). The owner reports that the animal has been anorexic for the last 24 hours. On clinical examination a right-sided head tilt is observed and, when placed on the floor, the animal exhibits a loss of equilibrium and falls to the right. There is no nystagmus present. Clinical examination is otherwise unremarkable.

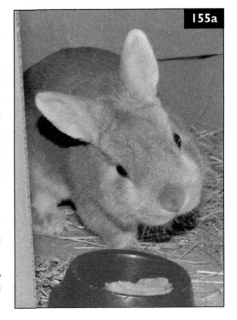

1 What are your differential diagnoses?
2 What further diagnostic tests are indicated?
3 What treatment options are there, and what is the long-term prognosis in this case?

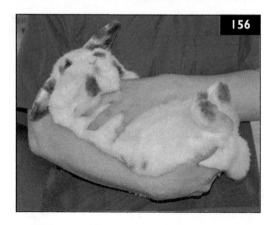

## CASE 156

1 What restraint technique is being used in this rabbit (156) and how is it achieved?
2 What procedures may be carried out using this technique?
3 What response is believed to underlie this behaviour?

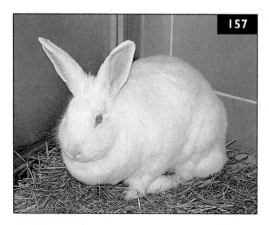

**CASE 157** An adult New Zealand White rabbit is presented with polyuria, polydypsia and glycosuria (157). Appetite and faecal output are reduced. Plasma biochemistry shows a raised blood glucose level of 16.2 mmol/l (normal reference range 4.2–8.3 mmol/l).

1 What is the likelihood of diabetes mellitus occurring in a pet rabbit?
2 How would you diagnose this condition?
3 What treatment would you commence in the event of diabetes mellitus being confirmed?

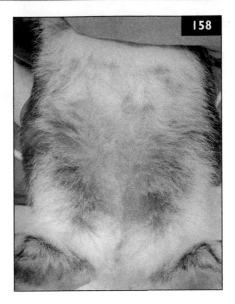

**CASE 158** An adult female entire Netherland Dwarf rabbit presents with fur pulling involving the ventral abdomen (**158**). The animal is housed indoors with another female rabbit.

1 What is the likely underlying condition?
2 What other clinical signs may be associated with this problem in does?
3 Why does this condition occur in the rabbit?
4 What are the treatment options available?

**CASE 159** A 10-week-old rabbit is presented for routine myxomatosis vaccination. On clinical examination you note this abnormality (**159**).

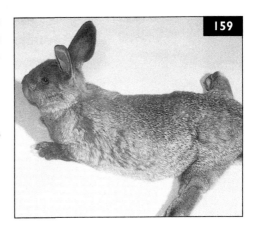

1 What is this condition?
2 What is the prognosis?
3 What advice should be given to the owner?

69

**CASE 160** A rabbit requires a pre-anaesthetic blood test.

1 How would you restrain a rabbit in order to take a jugular blood sample?
2 What are the risks of improper restraint?

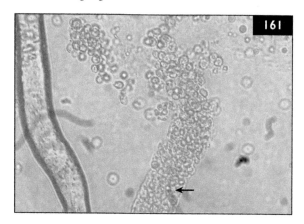

**CASE 161** These casts (161) were found in a urine sample, collected by cystocentesis, from a 6-year-old male rabbit.

1 What type of cast is shown?
2 Which type of cast, seen in dogs and cats, is almost never seen in rabbits, and why?
3 What is the significance of finding casts in rabbit urine?

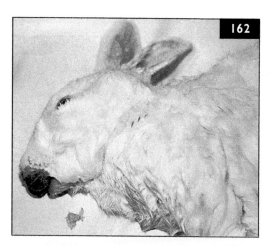

**CASE 162** This unvaccinated outdoor rabbit was found dead one morning (162). Blood was evident around the face. The rabbit had no previous signs of illness.

1 What are the possible causes of death in this animal?
2 What postmortem findings would confirm your diagnosis?

## CASE 163
1 What indications are there for the use of corticosteroids in rabbits?
2 What side effects may be seen when treating rabbits with corticosteroid drugs?

## CASE 164
1 What are the clinical signs associated with *Encephalitozoon cuniculi* infection in rabbits?
2 What diagnostic tests are available for confirming *E. cuniculi*?
3 What are the potential difficulties in reaching a definite diagnosis of active disease?

## CASE 165
1 What zoonotic organisms may be transmitted from rabbits?
2 What other health risk may rabbit owners face?

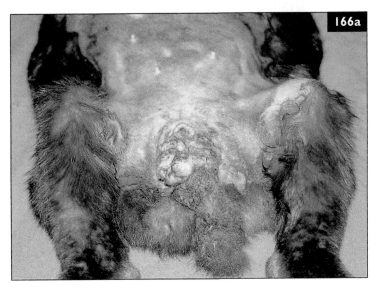

**CASE 166** A 5-year-old female French Lop rabbit has signs of urine scald of the perineum (**166a**). On clinical examination an excessive skin fold is observed surrounding the perineum. Describe both the medical and surgical treatment options in this case.

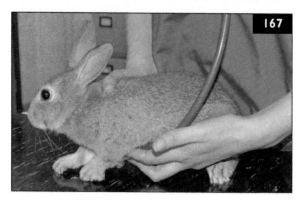

**CASE 167** An owner brings a 4-month-old rabbit to the veterinary practice for vaccination (167). What preventive health care topics should you discuss with the owner at this stage?

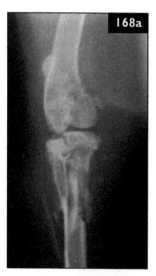

**CASE 168** A 1-year-old male entire rabbit, housed outdoors, is presented with a non-weight bearing lameness of the left hindlimb. The animal had been observed to be bright and well in the morning, but on the owner's return from work in the evening she found him to be depressed and reluctant to move. The distal half of the left hindlimb appeared rotated laterally. The rabbit was sedated and plain radiographs taken of the affected limb.

1 Describe the abnormality shown in the radiograph (168a).
2 What is the likely cause of the injury?
3 How could this problem be treated and managed?
4 What long-term considerations should be discussed with the owner following surgical treatment?

**CASE 169** Vaccination is advised in all domestic rabbits.

1 What viral infections are rabbits routinely vaccinated against in the UK?
2 Describe how the vaccination is administered and onset of immunity.
3 At what age can rabbits be vaccinated?
4 Are there any situations in which their use is contraindicated?

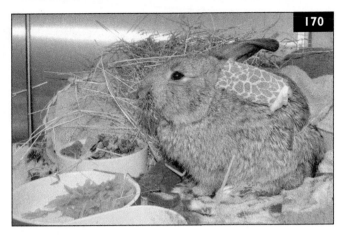

**CASE 170** This rabbit has a palpably enlarged liver (**170**). Which biochemical parameters may be used in the rabbit in the assessment of liver disease?

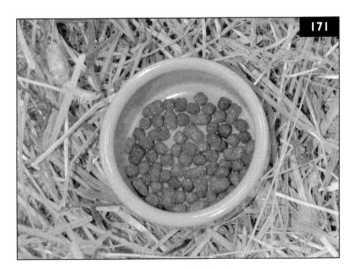

**CASE 171** An owner is concerned that her pet rabbit has ingested mouldy pellets. What potential toxin might these contain, and what clinical signs might it cause in the rabbit?

**CASE 172** What advice would you give an owner wishing to use preventive flea products on a pet rabbit?

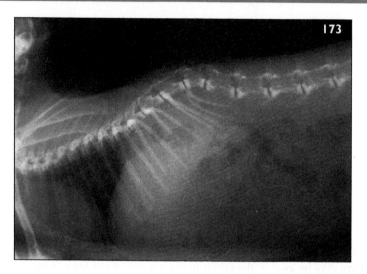

CASE 173 A 4-month-old male Netherland Dwarf rabbit is presented for assessment of a bilateral hindlimb weakness that has been apparent since the rabbit was acquired from a pet shop 6 weeks ago. The owner mentions that the rabbit occasionally appears to have poor balance and frequently falls over when grooming himself. The appetite is good and urination and faecal outputs are normal. On a physical and neurological examination the only abnormality detected is slow proprioceptive reflexes in both hindlimbs. The rabbit is anaesthetized and a series of spinal radiographs are taken, including the one shown (173).

1 Describe the abnormality.
2 What is the most likely cause of this problem?
3 What other diagnostic test could be performed to confirm the diagnosis?
4 Discuss treatment options.
5 What is the prognosis?

CASE 174 Which antibiotic drugs are known to be safe to use in rabbits, and by what route should they be administered?

CASE 175
1 What species of tick most commonly infects domestic rabbits?
2 For what diseases can ticks act as vectors?
3 How would you treat tick infection in a rabbit?

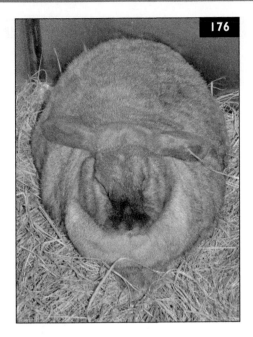

CASE 176 What secondary problems are associated with obesity in pet rabbits (176)?

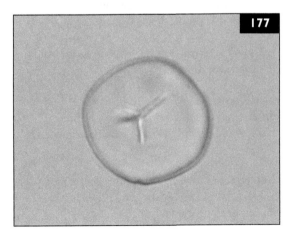

CASE 177 An object is observed on microscopic examination of a urine sample (177). It was collected immediately after a rabbit had its bladder expressed manually on the consultation table during a clinical examination. What is this object?

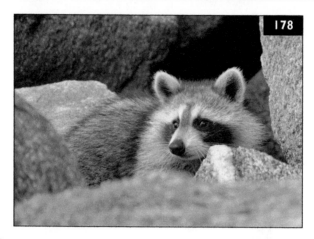

**CASE 178** A 1-year-old female spayed rabbit in the USA is housed outdoors with four other rabbits in a large enclosure with a wire mesh bottom. The rabbits are fed hay and pellets, which are stored in an open container in the owner's barn. The owner admits to having problems with raccoons (178) entering the barn and defecating in the area of food storage. Two of the other rabbits are displaying occasional tremors but this is the only rabbit with a head tilt.

1 How would you differentiate peripheral versus central disease in this rabbit?
2 List your differentials for a head tilt in a rabbit.
3 Given the history with this rabbit, what is the most likely cause of disease?

**CASE 179** An owner is worried that her rabbit's urine contains blood. She has brought in a urine sample for analysis.

1 How would you diagnose haematuria in the rabbit?
2 What are the differential diagnoses for this condition?
3 What further tests would you perform to reach a diagnosis?

**CASE 180** A rabbit presents with a 2-month history of progressive alopecia. There is considerable fur loss and scaling of the skin. The rabbit also displays bilateral exophthalmos with prominent third eyelids.

1 What is the most likely cause of the alopecia?
2 How would you confirm your diagnosis?
3 What treatment options are available?

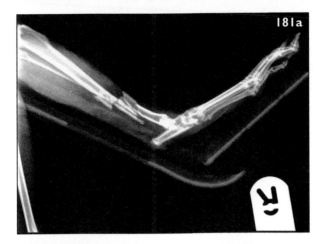

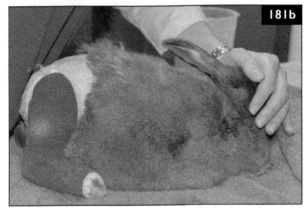

**CASE 181** Commercially available orthopaedic external fixator kits are useful and convenient for fracture fixation (**181a, b**) in many rabbits. However, in Dwarf or miniature breeds or juvenile animals this equipment may not be available in a suitable size.

1 What determines the maximum fixator pin diameter that should be used?
2 For smaller patients, what alternative materials can be used to construct external fixation that is equally rigid and resistant to chewing?
3 What factors affect the optimal time of removal of an external fixator in these patients?

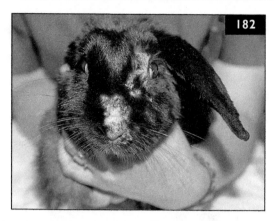

CASE 182 This rabbit is suffering from rabbit syphilis (182).

1 What is the causative agent, and how is it transmitted?
2 How is the condition diagnosed?
3 What treatment can be used?
4 What precautions should be taken when administering this drug to a rabbit?

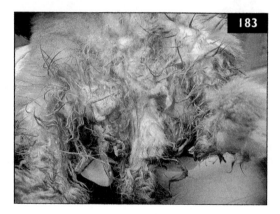

CASE 183 An adult female rabbit presents with urinary incontinence and secondary urine scalding of the perineum and medial aspect of the hindlimbs (183). What are your differential diagnoses?

CASE 184 The beneficial effects of probiotics in the prevention and treatment of rabbits with GI disease have been questioned in recent years. Why is this, and how are they thought to work in the rabbit?

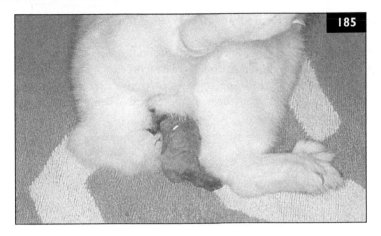

**CASE 185** You are presented with the rabbit shown (185).

1 What is your diagnosis?
2 What are the likely clinical signs associated with this condition?
3 What treatment options are available?

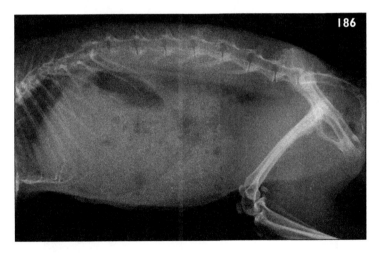

**CASE 186** This radiograph shows a lateral radiograph of the abdomen of a rabbit (186).

1 What abnormality can you detect?
2 What is the likely cause of this problem?
3 How would you treat it?

**CASE 187** A rabbit is in an incubator recovering from a general anaesthetic.

1  What are the key parameters that should be monitored?
2  With what frequency should parameters be recorded?
3  When would it be deemed appropriate to remove a recovering rabbit from an incubator or away from heat support, and when should postoperative monitoring cease?

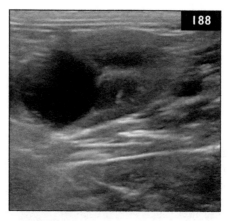

**CASE 188** On routine clinical examination of a 2-year-old pet rabbit an enlarged kidney is palpated. Ultrasound examination of the urogenital tract is performed.

1  Describe what you see in the ultrasound scan (**188**).
2  What is the clinical significance of this lesion, and what advice would you give to the owner?

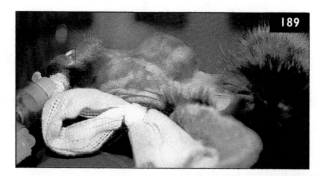

**CASE 189** This rabbit has a mandibular swelling that has been diagnosed as a dental abscess (**189**). How do you approach the treatment of dental abscesses?

**CASE 190** A 6-year-old rabbit is presented with chronic weight loss and polydypsia (190). The kidneys are palpably small. Serum biochemistry shows markedly elevated blood urea nitrogen (BUN), creatinine and phosphorus values and haematology reveals a non-regenerative anaemia. On urinalysis the urine is found to be isosthenuric. A diagnosis of chronic renal failure is made.

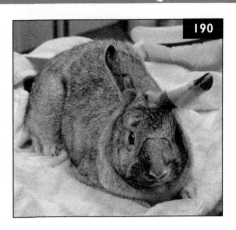

1 What can cause renal failure in rabbits?
2 How would you treat this condition?

**CASE 191**
1 To what secondary parasitic condition is this rabbit susceptible (191a)?
2 How would you treat an affected rabbit?
3 What husbandry advice would you give the owner?

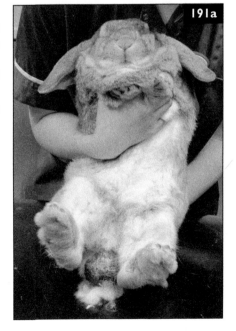

81

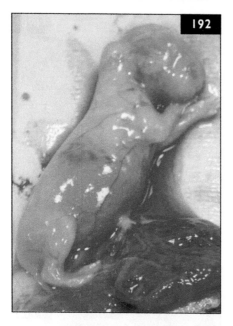

**CASE 192** A 1-year-old female rabbit has aborted at near term (**192**).

1 What are the possible causes?
2 How would you investigate this case?

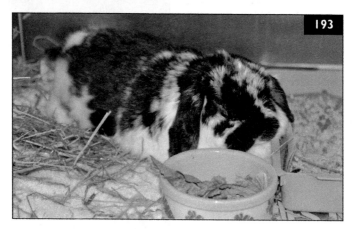

**CASE 193** A rabbit presented with a history of anorexia and mild depression following the death of its long-term companion (**193**). Faecal output had ceased. A radiograph of the abdomen showed the presence of gastric stasis and ileus.

1 How can non-obstructive and obstructive ileus be differentiated from each other?
2 How does their treatment differ?

## CASE 194

1 What condition is seen in this rabbit (194)?
2 List the predisposing factors to the development of this condition.
3 How would you treat it?

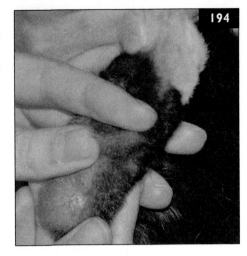

## CASE 195
A heavily gravid doe presents with anorexia, depression and collapse (195).

1 What is the likely diagnosis?
2 What is the prognosis?

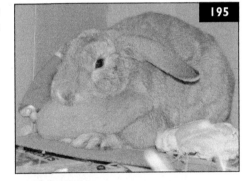

## CASE 196
An adult female entire rabbit is brought in for routine neutering. On clipping the fur, one of the mammary glands is found to be enlarged (196), although it does not appear hot or painful.

1 What are the differential diagnoses?
2 What further diagnostic tests are indicated?
3 What treatment is indicated?

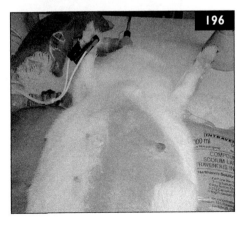

**CASE 197** Name two poxvirus skin diseases of rabbits. For each one, describe the natural host and the clinical signs in both the natural host and the domestic rabbit.

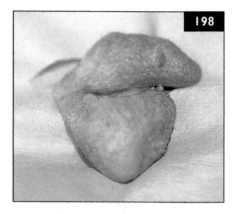

**CASE 198** A 1-year-old entire male rabbit is presented with an enlarged testicle (**198**).

1  What are the differential diagnoses?
2  What is the treatment of choice?

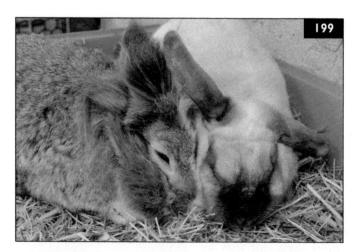

**CASE 199** What standard procedures should be considered prior to euthanasia in pet rabbits (**199**)?

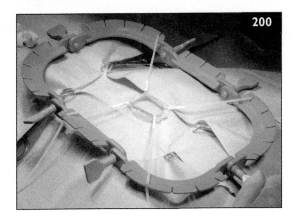

**CASE 200** Rabbits are extremely prone to ileus and adhesion formation following abdominal surgery (200). What surgical precautions should be taken to reduce the risk of these conditions developing in the postoperative period?

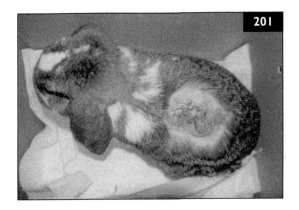

**CASE 201** A 6-month-old male rabbit that is housed with another entire male of the same age is shown (201). An area of skin on the dorsum is reddened and swollen with patchy scabbing. The rabbit is lethargic and partially anorexic. What is the most likely cause of this lesion, and how would you treat it?

**CASE 202**
1  Describe the surgical techniques used to castrate male rabbits.
2  What is the minimum recommended time post surgery that a male rabbit should be separated from its intact female companion?

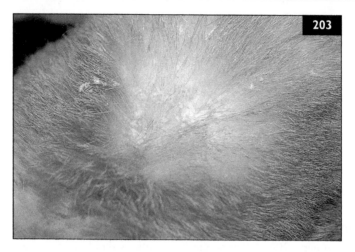

## CASE 203

1 What ectoparasite is generally associated with these clinical signs (203)?
2 How would you treat this animal?
3 Are there any zoonotic implications?

**CASE 204** What are the differential diagnoses for alopecia in the rabbit?

**CASE 205** A 6-month-old female neutered Netherland Dwarf rabbit is presented for assessment of a right forelimb lameness of 4 days' duration. The owner reports that the rabbit, a normally flighty individual, escaped from her hutch on the morning that the injury was first noticed, although no traumatic incident was observed. On examination the rabbit is non-weight bearing on the right forelimb, there is an open wound on the medial aspect of the limb 1 cm (0.4 inch) distal to the elbow and a smaller puncture wound on the lateral aspect at the same level. There is marked crepitus on flexion and extension of the right elbow, and at full extension a small fragment of discoloured bone is visible at the edge of the medial wound. The owners have strict financial limitations but are reluctant to consider euthanasia.

1 What is the treatment of choice, and what factors influence this decision?
2 What is the prognosis?
3 Discuss pre- and postoperative considerations in such a case.
4 What equipment would be required for the surgery?

**CASE 206** What reflexes may be used in the assessment of anaesthetic depth in the rabbit?

**CASE 207** A 7-year-old entire female Dutch rabbit, housed indoors, presents with weight loss, anorexia and acute-onset severe dyspnoea and rapid fatigue. The rabbit is thin, alert but weak. Mucous membranes are cyanotic but capillary refill time and pulse are normal. Abdominal palpation is tense. Lung sounds are generally decreased. There is a poor response to oxygen therapy. Lateral and dorsoventral radiographs are shown (**207a, b**).

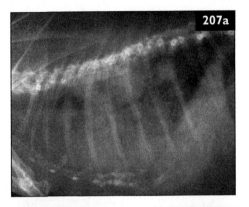

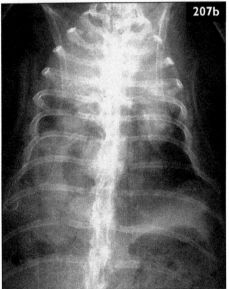

1 What radiographic changes are present and what is the most likely diagnosis given the signalment and clinical signs?
2 What differential diagnoses would you consider in a 7-year-old rabbit with these clinical signs?
3 What is the prognosis?
4 What preventive measures are there to reduce the incidence of this condition?

**CASE 208** A 2-year-old anorexic rabbit is hospitalized for nutritional support. What techniques and preparations can be used to administer oral nutritional support in the rabbit?

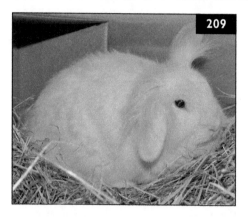

**CASE 209** A 2-year-old female neutered rabbit kept outdoors is presented with non-specific clinical signs of weight loss and anorexia. On abdominal palpation a grossly enlarged spleen is palpable (209). What are your main differential diagnoses for splenomegaly in this rabbit?

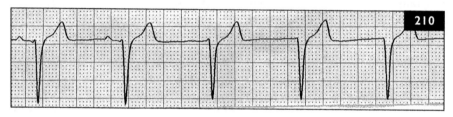

**CASE 210** An electrocardiogram from a 5-year-old male Lop rabbit with an intermittent heart rate of 200 beats per minute (bpm) is shown (210). The rabbit showed episodic weakness associated with the arrhythmia, which lasted for 20–30 beats every few hours.

1 What is your diagnosis?
2 How would you treat this condition?

**CASE 211** A 3-year-old entire female rabbit has been anorexic and lethargic for 12 hours. Increased tympany is evident on abdominal percussion. A mass is palpable in the mid-abdomen.

1 What differential diagnoses are there for an intestinal mass?
2 What further investigative techniques would you use to reach a diagnosis?
3 In this rabbit, a caecal intussusception is diagnosed. Gastric and small intestinal dilatation was present on abdominal radiography, suggesting an obstruction. Blood glucose was 22 mmol/l. Describe the management of this case.

## CASE 212

1 What are these structures in the inguinal region (212)?
2 Where are similar structures also found in the rabbit, and what is their purpose?
3 How do they differ between the sexes?

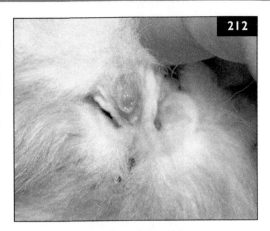

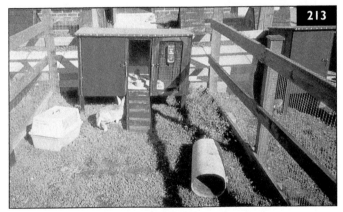

**CASE 213** A purpose-built outdoor enclosure containing a hutch is shown (213). Evaluate this housing arrangement for a rabbit, noting the important features and their relevance.

**CASE 214** A 5-year-old female entire Dutch rabbit presented with red discolouration of the urine. A caudal abdominal mass was evident on abdominal palpation. Abdominal radiographs showed a normal intestinal tract and urinary tract, with a mass of soft tissue density in the region of the uterus. Ultrasonography confirmed the mass to be an enlarged uterus.

1 What are your differential diagnoses?
2 How would you manage this case?
3 What is the prognosis?

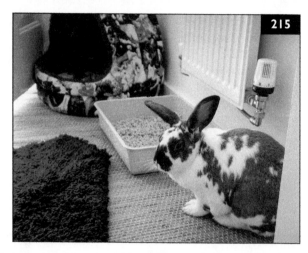

**CASE 215** A 2-year-old male rabbit has started urinating outside its litter tray and is soiling the furniture within the home. The rabbit has been neutered and it was trained to use the tray from an early age (**215**). The owner has tried to change the brand of litter and moved the tray but the problem persists. What could be the possible behavioural causes of this problem, and how can they be addressed?

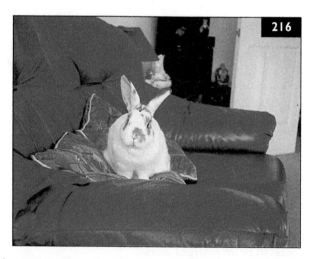

**CASE 216** House rabbits are now very popular pets (**216**). What provisions should be made for their accommodation, to ensure their safety and to minimize mess and damage to the house?

CASE 217 An owner wishes to medicate his/her pet rabbit at home. What advice can you give to facilitate the administration of an oral medication?

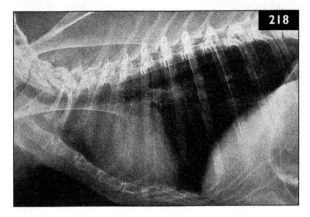

CASE 218 A lateral thoracic radiograph from a pet rabbit is shown (218). What normal anatomical features can be seen?

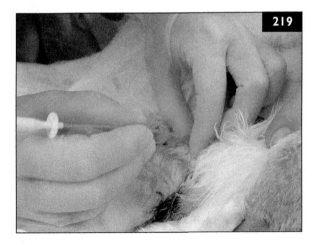

CASE 219
1 What examination technique is being shown (219)?
2 What conditions may be diagnosed using this technique?

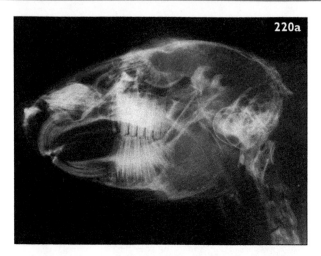

**CASE 220** What procedure is shown in this lateral radiograph of a rabbit's skull (220a)? Describe how this is carried out and in what circumstances it is indicated.

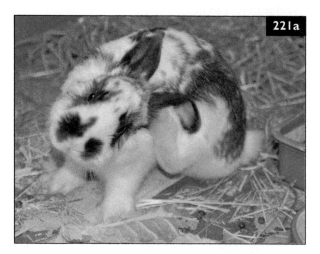

**CASE 221** This rabbit presented with a history of head shaking and scratching of the pinnae (221a).

1 What organism is most likely to be causing the clinical signs and lesions?
2 How would you confirm your diagnosis?
3 How might the lesions progress?
4 What treatment is appropriate?

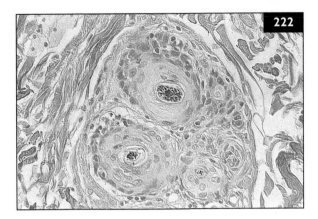

**CASE 222** This rabbit presented with generalized non-pruritic scaling and alopecia. Diagnostic tests excluded ectoparasites, dermatophytes, yeasts and bacteria as causative agents.

1 What disease is shown in the histological section (**222**)?
2 What treatment may be attempted?

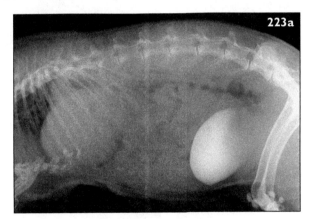

**CASE 223** A 2-year-old male neutered rabbit presents with weight loss, urine scalding and anorexia. On clinical examination abdominal palpation is resented and the rabbit exhibits bruxism (teeth grinding). A radiograph is taken (**223a**).

1 What is your diagnosis?
2 What further diagnostic tests would you perform?
3 What treatment is indicated?
4 What preventive measures would you instigate?

93

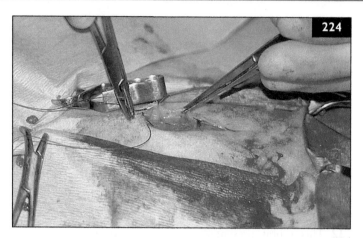

**CASE 224** What volume of blood constitutes a critical blood loss in a rabbit undergoing a surgical procedure (**224**)?

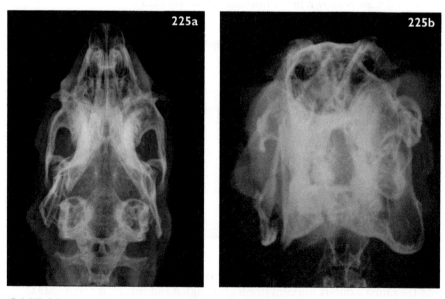

**CASE 225** A rabbit presents subdued and inappetant after being free-range out in the garden. The owner reports that the rabbit is having difficulty eating. You decide to take dorsoventral and rostrocaudal skull radiographs (**225a, b**). Describe your findings and possible treatment options.

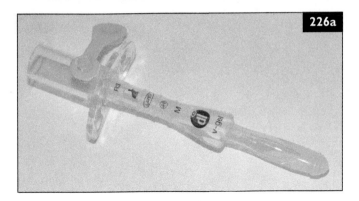

**CASE 226** Supraglottic airway devices can be used to supply inhalation anaesthetic maintenance in rabbits (**226a**).

1 Describe what this device is and how it works.
2 What are the advantages and disadvantages of supraglottic airway devices?

**CASE 227** Describe how you would collect a sample using a bronchoalveolar lavage technique.

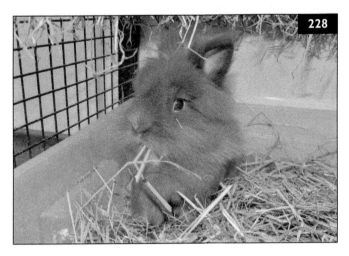

**CASE 228** Pineapple juice is often used by owners to treat and prevent hairball formation. Is this a treatment you would recommend to owners?

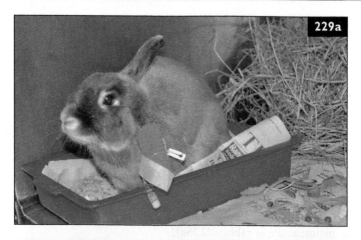

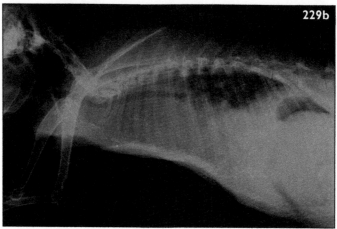

**CASE 229** A rabbit presents in severe respiratory distress (**229a**). After oxygen therapy, a conscious lateral thoracic radiograph was obtained using a horizontal beam (**229b**).

1 Discuss the thoracic radiographic findings.
2 Based on the radiographic findings, what procedure would be beneficial to the patient?
3 What is the likely prognosis in this case?

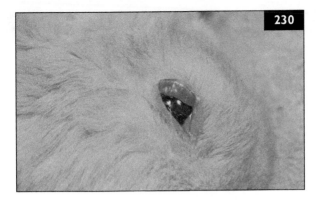

**CASE 230** At a routine health check you notice several raised lesions on the conjunctiva of the upper eyelid (**230**).

1  What are these lesions?
2  What treatment would you advise to the owner?

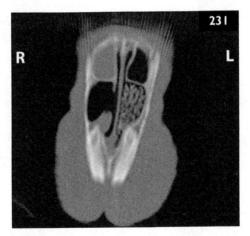

**CASE 231** A rabbit presents subdued with a unilateral nasal discharge that has been unresponsive to a 10-day course of enrofloxacin. The client declines radiography and rhinoscopy and opts for a conscious CT scan to assess the respiratory system. Lung fields appear normal, but abnormalities are noted in the nasal passage (**231**).

1  Discuss the findings from this rostral cross-section image taken at the level of the upper incisors.
2  What is your diagnosis?

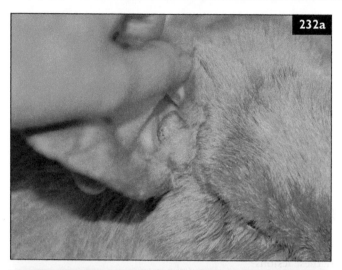

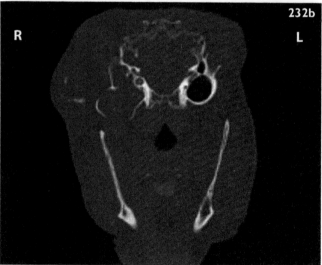

CASE 232 An elderly rabbit presents with a polyp in the external ear canal (232a). On physical examination pus is visible proximal to the polyp. The owner also reports recent concerns over a reduction in the rabbit's hearing. You perform a CT scan to assess the auditory system. Describe the changes seen at the level of the tympanic bulla (232b).

# CASE 1
Describe the techniques available for endotracheal intubation of an anaesthetized rabbit (1a, b, c, d).

1 *Direct visualization.* Place the anaesthetized rabbit in sternal recumbency, extend the neck vertically by elevating the head, grasp the tongue gently and retract it through the diastema and hold to one side. Visualize the larynx using a Wisconsin size 1 laryngoscope blade (**1a**) and insert a 2.5–3.0 mm endotracheal tube (**1b**). Alternatively, position the rabbit as above, visualize the larynx using an otoscope or Wisconsin size 1 laryngoscope blade or similar, place an introducer (e.g. 3–5 Fr urinary catheter) into the larynx through an otoscope or over a laryngoscope, remove the otoscope/laryngoscope and introduce an endotracheal tube gently over the introducer and then remove the introducer. A further alternative is to use the otoscope and place the endotracheal tube with its connector removed directly through the otoscope cone, replacing the connector after removal of the otoscope. The larynx can also be visualized using a small rigid endoscope while the endotracheal tube is passed alongside it into the larynx.

All the above methods can also be performed with the rabbit in dorsal recumbency with the neck extended.

2 *Blind technique.* Hold the anaesthetized rabbit in sternal recumbency with the head and neck extended. Pass an endotracheal tube over the tongue and advance it until exhalation is heard loudly either by placing the end of the tube to the ear (**1c**) or by the presence of condensation at each breath if using a clear tube, then advance the tube gently as the rabbit inhales and it will pass into the trachea.

For all these techniques, positioning is important. Rabbits are obligate nasal breathers so normally the epiglottis is engaged on the dorsal aspect of the soft palate and will require disengagement in order to gain access to the glottal opening via the mouth. As with many techniques, there are several options and personal preferences. The author prefers to extend the neck vertically with no weight on the forelimbs. The neck is fully extended by holding the back of the rabbit's head and elevating this. Insertion of the laryngoscope or otoscope is generally all that is required to disengage the epiglottis from the soft palate and expose the glottis (**1d**). If using a rigid endoscope, gentle dorsal pressure on the soft palate will dislodge the epiglottis. The anaesthetized rabbit should be allowed to breathe 100% oxygen by mask for a few minutes before intubation is attempted. With all these techniques, never force the tube into the larynx as this will cause haemorrhage and oedema and increase the risk of laryngospasm. A good rule is to make three attempts only and, if unsuccessful, revert to a mask. Topical lidocaine spray applied to the larynx may be used. This can be done under direct visualization with a spray. Some practitioners prefer to insert the tube blind to the level of the larynx and trickle or gently blow a few drops of lidocaine down the inside of the tube on to the larynx.

An alternative to endotracheal intubation is to use a laryngeal mask (see case 226).

## CASE 2

**1 Describe what can be seen (2a).** The fundus picture shows marked cupping of the optic disc and retinal vessel attenuation. This may be compared with the merangiotic fundus of the normal rabbit eye **(2b)**. This is a result of loss of optic nerve fibres due to progressive glaucoma. Glaucoma is hereditary in New Zealand White rabbits,

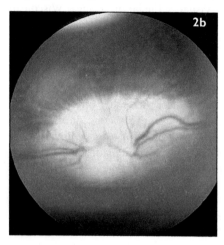

associated with the recessive *bu* gene, but it can also be secondary to severe uveitis or intraocular neoplasia. The blindness will not have been a sudden occurrence but will have been present prior to the change of housing, the rabbit coping well with its limited environment.

**2 What is the prognosis in this case?** The prognosis for restoration of vision is nil but, provided the rabbit can be encouraged to learn its way around the run and can find and compete for food successfully, it can lead a satisfactory life. Medical treatment for primary glaucoma is rarely effective or necessary.

## CASE 3

**1 What is the definition of obesity?** An excessive accumulation of fat in the body. This occurs when the energy intake exceeds the energy expenditure. As a guideline, any rabbit whose body weight is more than 20% above that considered desirable for their age, breed and build is likely to be obese. Obese rabbits will have a body condition score of 5 (on a scale of 1–5) where it is very hard or impossible to palpate the spine, ribs and pelvic bones due to subcutaneous fat deposition, heavy deposits of adipose tissue over the neck and upper limbs, and abdominal distension due to extensive intra-abdominal fat deposits.

**2 How would you achieve weight loss in this rabbit?** The eventual aim would be to convert this rabbit to a diet based on *ad libitum* provision of good quality hay, access to grass and fresh weeds, a daily serving of mixed fresh greens and a very limited amount of high-fibre homogeneous extruded nuggets or pellets. Mixed rations (muesli-type mixes) have been demonstrated to lead directly to obesity in rabbits when fed without *ad libitum* hay, as well as being associated with dental disease, reduced gastrointestinal motility and behavioural changes.

It is important, however, to realize that weight loss must be gradual (no more than 1–2% of body weight weekly) and great care should be taken from the outset to prevent periods of anorexia (e.g. by offering an unfamiliar diet), as this may lead to the development of hepatic lipidosis. Any sudden change of diet must also be avoided, as this can cause serious disturbance to the intestinal microflora and dysbiosis. Owner compliance is paramount in any pet weight loss plan, so discussions regarding the challenge ahead and setting achievable goals are important from the outset.

The first change to make is to ensure that good quality hay is offered *ad libitum*. The concentrate ration should be slowly reduced from the diet over a period of a few weeks, until it is eliminated completely. Mixed fresh greens can be given daily unless gastrointestinal upset occurs and the yoghurt/carob drops, table scraps and other treats should be removed from the diet. If normal body condition is achieved, it may be possible or desirable to add a very small amount of homogeneous extruded pellets back into the maintenance ration.

Most obese rabbits are largely inactive. To complement dietary changes, increasing activity levels by encouraging play time, providing environmental enrichment and/or allowing access to large outdoor runs or escape-proof gardens is a key component of any weight loss programme.

## CASE 4

**1 Describe how this is performed.** This procedure requires the rabbit to be anaesthetized. A fine swab is premeasured to the level of the medial canthus of the eye from the external nares. This is introduced into the ventral nasal cavity and advanced slowly in a ventromedial direction. Iatrogenic damage to the nasal turbinates is common. Unless care is taken, contaminants are common from the external nares. Both sides should be sampled for comparison.

**2 What alternative method could be employed?** An alternative is to use nasal endoscopy. A small (1.9 mm) rigid endoscope can be inserted into the nares to visualize the nasal cavity and obtain mucosal biopsies which can be submitted for both culture and histopathology. This method is preferable as there is direct visualization and less likelihood of contamination.

**3 What is the significance of a mixed bacterial culture being obtained?** A pure single culture is likely to be clinically significant; a mixed culture probably represents normal bacterial flora. Bacteria found in normal nasal flora in healthy rabbits include *Moraxella catarrhalis*, *Bordetella bronchiseptica*, *Pasteurella multocida*, *Staphylococcus* spp., *Streptococcus* spp. and *Bacillus* spp.

## CASE 5

**Why is mask induction with a volatile anaesthetic agent risky in an unsedated rabbit (5)?** Due to their prey status, rabbits are very easily stressed. They are also prone to prolonged breath holding and bradycardia when in contact with volatile anaesthetic agents. Firm restraint is generally required in an unsedated rabbit, as the animal will resent the face mask and agent and will struggle, risking spinal injury, and high stress levels. Breath holding may go unnoticed and the induction concentration may be increased to high levels before a breath is taken, resulting in sudden inspiration of a high concentration. Stress will increase circulating catecholamines and there will be an increased risk of cardiac arrest, especially if halothane is used. If mask induction is used, the rabbit must be monitored closely and the face mask removed if breath holding occurs and replaced when breathing recommences. It is preferable to use a tranquillizer or sedative prior to induction. This will not prevent breath holding but will minimize stress and prevent excessive struggling.

## CASE 6

**1 What are the differential diagnoses in this case?** Congestive heart failure (myocardial, valvular and congenital disease) is seen in middle-aged to older rabbits. The weakness, weight loss and rapid fatigue observed, although non-specific signs, should arouse suspicion of cardiac or lower respiratory disease. Other differentials include: pyothorax – pleuropneumonia typically due to pasteurellosis but other bacterial agents are often involved; modified transudates seen secondary to neoplasia, lung lobe torsion or diaphragmatic hernia; haemothorax – seen in viral haemorrhagic disease, coagulopathies or trauma.

**2 Based on the radiographic findings, what immediate treatment would you consider?** The radiographs show a pleural effusion. Immediate thoracocentesis will help stabilize the rabbit as well as determine the type of effusion. Drain the thorax bilaterally using a 23 gauge butterfly catheter placed ventrally in the chest wall. Remove as much fluid as possible by aspirating multiple sites. Oxygen should be provided via a face mask during this procedure and stress should be kept to a minimum. Sedation is often not required in debilitated animals, although diazepam (0.5–1 mg/kg i/v or i/m) or midazolam (1–2 mg/kg i/v or i/m) may be used if necessary. In this case 20 ml of a serosanguinous fluid was obtained from both left and right sides of the chest. It was found to be a modified transudate with a protein of 22.4 g/l (ref: 25–30 g/l) and a nucleated cell count of $2 \times 10^9$/l (ref: $1–7 \times 10^9$/l). No organisms were cultured.

**3 What further diagnostic tests might be helpful?** Once the rabbit is stable the thoracic radiography is repeated to evaluate fully the thoracic contents. Echocardiography should be carried out to characterize any cardiac disease further. Electrocardiography, blood pressure measurement and routine blood tests are useful in reaching a definitive diagnosis and treatment plan.

## CASE 7

**What advice would you give the owners regarding this destructive behaviour?**
Ideally, this rabbit should be living in the home full-time if the owners desire this as the outcome, but there are several factors to address. The first is puberty, which occurs from about 4 months of age in dwarf breeds. It is probable that this rabbit's intermittent toileting is a consequence of his need to mark areas with his scent, particularly as he is not in the home that often. If the rabbit is also exhibiting inappropriate sexual behaviour, neutering should be discussed with the owner.

Rabbits that live in the home should have an area that they can retreat to, so an indoor cage would be an appropriate purchase. The owners should place the litter tray in this location, as well as his food. If necessary, the rabbit can be confined in this area for a period of 3–4 days to help establish appropriate toilet training. A dog exercise pen that consists of removable wire panels is a useful method of providing a safe exercise area indoors.

The destructive behaviour is quite normal in an animal that grazes to obtain its food. The owners should be advised to rethink the rabbit's diet to ensure that he is spending more time obtaining food than at present. The emphasis should be on good quality hay making up the bulk of the diet and being used in foraging exercises. The owners can be encouraged to fill toys with hay or to introduce a hayrack. In addition, a small quantity of green vegetables and extruded nugget or pellet can be fed to the rabbit. Fresh fruit should be regarded as an occasional treat item only.

To avoid inappropriate learning and a fearful response, the owners should be encouraged not to reprimand the rabbit for the destructive behaviour. When the rabbit first comes into the home, he should initially be given access to small areas so that he can be supervised and also offered toys, old cardboard boxes, inner tubes of kitchen rolls and egg boxes to chew as an alternative. Filling them with hay or food can encourage interest in these items.

## CASE 8

**1 What are the main abnormalities?** Pancytopenia, hypoproteinaemia and uraemia.
**2 What is the likely cause?** Renal failure. Decreased erythropoietin production leads to a non-regenerative anaemia. Bone marrow suppression associated with chronic disease occurs commonly in rabbits. With results like these, where all the haematology parameters are low, a dilution artefact, such as flushing a syringe with heparin-saline before taking a small volume blood sample, should be considered. This is unlikely in this case, since although some biochemistry results are low, urea is elevated. If in doubt, haematology and biochemistry should be repeated. Low proteins may be due to a renal protein loss. Serum creatinine levels have not been evaluated, but urea is elevated and azotaemia is likely.

**3 How may this be confirmed?** Serum creatinine levels should be evaluated to confirm an azotaemia. Urine specific gravity (SG) determined with a refractometer and proteinurea evaluated on urine dipsticks will help determine if the azotaemia is of renal origin. Isosthenuric urine may indicate a loss of tubular function. While trace proteins may be present in normal rabbit urine, this should be evaluated in conjunction with the SG. Proteinuria is relatively more important when detected in dilute urine. It is possible to evaluate the degree of proteinuria further by calculating the urine protein to creatinine ratio, which should normally be <1.0. Examination of urine for casts can also be useful – cellular and granular casts are indicative of renal damage. Hyaline casts are not normally found in rabbits due to their alkaline urine.

## CASE 9
**1 Describe the findings shown by lead II of the electrocardiogram.** Normal sinus rhythm.
**2 What treatment is indicated?** While the rabbit is hospitalized, provide treatment with oxygen therapy, repeated therapeutic thoracocentesis if dyspnoeic, parenteral frusemide (furosemide) (1–4 mg/kg i/v or i/m q4–12h) and nitroglycerine 2% ointment (3 mm [1/8 inch] applied transdermally q6–12h). Long-term therapy with positive inotropic agents such as digoxin (3–30 ug/kg p/o q24–48h) and antihypertensive drugs (e.g. benazepril 0.05 mg/kg p/o q24h) as appropriate should be directed at the underlying disease.
**3 What is the prognosis?** Prognosis will depend on the response to treatment.

## CASE 10
**1 Identify the indicated organism. Why is this staining not what one would expect?** *Clostridium spiriforme*. This bacterium often has a c-shaped appearance. Clostridia are Gram-positive, endospore-forming bacteria, but they decolorize easily with Gram's stain solvents (ethanol or acetone-ethanol) and so often stain falsely Gram negative.
**2 Is this organism a normal part of the rabbit enteric flora?** No. While some authors believe *C. spiriforme* is a normal commensal found in very low numbers, its appearance on faecal smears is not regarded as normal. Little is known about the transmission of *C. spiriforme*.
**3 What specific requirements are needed for isolating this organism?** Anaerobic bacterial culture methods are needed. Standard culture media such a blood agar or a selective media such as Mackonkey blood agar are adequate for isolation.

**4 What causes the clinical signs seen?** Clostridial enterotoxaemia is acute or peracute in onset. A pet rabbit may appear normal in the evening and be found dead the next morning. *C. spiriforme* produces an iota-like enterotoxin in the caecum, which causes enteric damage, dehydration and electrolyte imbalance to occur. Clinical signs when seen consist of lethargy and a green-brown diarrhoea. Death usually ensues within 48 hours.

**5 What factors predispose to the development of clostridial enterotoxaemia?** Diet is important; rabbits on a high-fibre, hay- or grass-based diet are much less likely to develop clostridial enterotoxaemia than rabbits on a cereal-mix based diet, which is high in refined carbohydrates. Refined or easily fermentable carbohydrates lead to a lower caecal pH than normal, which is a more suitable environment for clostridial multiplication. Antibiotic use is another important factor. Clindamycin, lincomycin and erythromycin are contraindicated in rabbits, as their selective effect on Gram-positive bacteria will lead to *Clostridium* spp. overgrowth and enterotoxaemia. The same applies to orally administered penicillins and cephalosporins, which can result in an incidence of up to 80% enterotoxaemia after administration. In young rabbits, preventing stress at the time of weaning is helpful in preventing the occurrence of this condition. Stress is believed to predispose to enterotoxaemia by the release of catecholamines reducing normal gut motility.

## CASE 11

**1 What are the potential benefits of spaying does, and what is the recommended age for this procedure?** Unwanted pregnancy and pseudopregnancy will be prevented. Territorial aggression is often reduced, as it may be a sexually related behaviour. Uterine neoplasia, particularly adenocarcinoma, is common in entire does and ovariohysterectomy is recommended before 2 years old to reduce the incidence of this condition. Pyometra may also occur in intact female rabbits and is prevented by this surgical procedure. Spayed does can live with bucks (preferably castrated). The average recommended age for neutering female rabbits is from 5 months onwards and before 2 years old.

**2 Describe the surgical technique of ovariohysterectomy in the rabbit.** The anaesthetized rabbit is placed in dorsal recumbency. The caudal abdomen is clipped and prepared aseptically. A small midline incision made anterior to the pubis in line with the caudal abdominal nipples will provide good exposure of the reproductive tract. The vaginal body is located as a relatively large flaccid structure dorsal to the bladder. Because the Fallopian tubes are friable, gentle traction only should be applied to the uterine horns to exteriorize the ovaries. Obese rabbits will have large amounts of fat in the mesovarium and mesometrium, making ovarian location and visualization of blood vessels difficult, and they should preferably lose weight prior to surgery. Place ligatures (absorbable mono- or multifilament synthetic suture material) across the ovarian blood vessels and those in the mesometrium. Ligate the cervices by applying a length of suture material around each uterine horn before encompassing the cervical region/cervical body; once tightened this ligature sits securely across both cervices without the need to transfix the vagina and prevents urine leakage from the vagina. To achieve this individually, encompass and tie off each horn at the bifurcation by passing the suture material through a puncture in the mesometrium so it encircles the base of one horn, tie the ligature but do not cut it, and pass the same suture material to encircle the contralateral horn base (again tie but do not cut); finally, take the ligature around the body encompassing the entire cervical area, tighten, knot and cut.

Alternatively, the uterine horns may be removed by ligating either cranial or caudal to the cervices (**11**). If using a cranial transfixing ligature, there is no risk of urine contamination of the abdomen from the uterus; however, a small amount of uterine tissue may remain with the potential to develop adenocarcinomatous changes at a future date. Once the ovaries have been removed, the risk is small. If a caudal ligature is used, care should be taken to avoid contamination of the abdomen with urine or vaginal contents during surgery, since the urethra of the female rabbit empties into the proximal vaginal vestibule. The vaginal stump can be oversewn with a continuous inverting suture layer of monofilament absorbable suture material in order to minimize this risk. There is a small risk if using the caudal ligature technique that damage to the vessels supplying the bladder may occur while placing the ligature, or that the ureters may be included in the ligature if it is placed too far caudally.

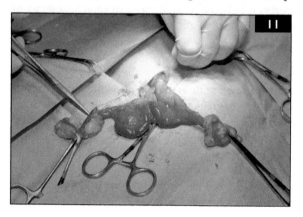

**3 Are there any alternatives to surgical ovariohysterectomy?** Ovariectomy, achieved via conventional surgical techniques or via laparoscopy, is an alternative, particularly in young rabbits. This is quicker, requires a much smaller incision and avoids potential complications from ligature placement close to the bladder and ureters. The likelihood of remaining uterine tissue undergoing neoplastic change is not known but there are no published reports. In older rabbits (over 1 year) ovariohysterectomy is generally recommended due to the risk of uterine pathology.

## CASE 12

**1 What is the lesion shown?** This is a hemivertebra, a congenital malformation of the spine.

**2 What surgical treatment option is available?** If the neurological change is progressive, a decompressive laminectomy with stabilization of the spine may prevent further deterioration. There are no published reports of this procedure in pet rabbits but anecdotal reports exist and it is described as a research technique.

## CASE 13

**Identify the organs labelled 1–6 on this rabbit abdomen (13).** (1) Stomach; (2) liver; (3) left kidney; (4) caecum; (5) proximal colon; (6) small intestine.

## CASE 14

**Describe placement of a urethral catheter to obtain a urine sample in a buck rabbit (14).** Catheterization of male rabbits is relatively straightforward but urethrospasm is commonly encountered. This may be avoided by prior administration of dipyrone/hyoscine and application of a sterile local anaesthetic gel to the catheter tip. The patient is sedated and positioned in either dorsal recumbency with the thorax elevated or lateral recumbency. Sterile gloves should be worn. The penis is everted and a sterile lubricated urinary 3–4 Fr gauge feline urinary catheter is advanced gently into the urethral opening. Some resistance may be felt as the catheter passes through the urethra as it courses over the pelvic brim. Urine should be visible in the catheter if placement is successful and a 5–10 ml syringe can be attached to aspirate urine.

## CASE 15

**1 What are the radiographic findings?** The radiograph shows increased opacity on the right side of the nasal cavity.

**2 What additional diagnostic tests can be performed to better define the problem?** Advance imaging techniques such as endoscopy, CT scan or MRI are indicated in this case. Endoscopy requires general anaesthesia and allows direct visualization of the nasal cavity and the collection of samples and biopsies. However, unless there is major destruction of the turbinates/conchae, endoscopy of the most caudal aspect of the nasal cavity is generally complicated. CT scan (and also MRI) can be performed under mild sedation or, in some cases, with no sedation at all.

Considering the generalized increased opacity revealed on radiography, a CT scan was performed in this case and this revealed complete atrophy of the ventral nasal conchae of the right nasal cavity and the presence of purulent material completely filling the right maxillary sinus and partially filling the right frontal sinus.

**3 How would you treat this case?** Considering both the chronic clinical history and the results of computer tomography, it is unlikely that medical treatment will resolve this case. The purulent material that has accumulated in the sinuses needs to be physically removed or the infection will continue destroying the nasal structures. In addition, rabbit pus tends to become caseous with time and antibiotic treatment is usually unsuccessful at this stage. The treatment of choice in this case is to perform a dorsal rhinotomy, opening a hole in the right nasal bone and using it to collect samples and to remove any secretions and debride abnormal tissues. The affected nasal cavity is then flushed rostrally and the skin over the bony defect is closed routinely. Periodic flushing can be continued by aseptically inserting a needle attached to a saline-filled syringe through the skin over the defect; alternatively, a catheter can be sutured in placed at the time of surgery and flushing with warm sterile saline continued for several days to weeks, until the clinical signs disappear.

## CASE 16

**1 Describe the method you would use.** Examination of the rabbit's oral cavity is the most difficult part of any clinical examination but is essential and should be performed routinely. Rabbits do not like their mouth being touched and often resent any attempts to examine the teeth. Owners should always be warned of the limitations of conscious oral examination and that abnormalities are easily missed. The rabbit is restrained on the examination table by an assistant, or the owner, who holds it around the shoulders. The hindquarters are tucked in towards the assistant's abdomen and the rabbit faces away from them. In fractious animals a towel may be used to wrap around the animal, although this is rarely required. The veterinary surgeon is now free to hold the rabbit's head with one hand and use the other hand to examine the mouth. The lips and jaws should be palpated for any deformities or swellings. If in pain, the rabbit may resent palpation of these areas. The lips should be retracted to examine the incisors, the interdigital area and the buccal mucosa. The mandible should be manipulated laterally while stabilizing the maxilla to assess if there is any inhibition of normal lateral movement, or any pain associated with such movement. An otoscope or canine vaginal speculum with light source may be gently inserted into the mouth, allowing visualization of the cheek teeth, interdigital area, hard palate and tongue. An alternative method of restraint for oral examination of a conscious rabbit is to scruff it and turn it on to its back. This should always be carried out over an examination table and by experienced personnel. This may be a stressful experience if the rabbit is not conditioned to being handled in this way.

**2 Can an accurate dental assessment be made?** Chemical restraint is needed for a more detailed oral examination. Specialist incisor gags and cheek pouch retractors, combined with good illumination and/or magnification with ocular loops, are necessary. Alternatively, a rigid endoscope may be used.

## CASE 17

**What advice would you give?** There are two areas to address here: the digging and the choice of companion. In the wild, female rabbits start to dig scrapes and burrows at the beginning of the breeding season (late January). The behaviour diminishes during the autumn and winter. This response to the seasons is still present in domestic rabbits and explains the intermittent behaviour exhibited by this case. Neutering might help solve the problem, but the introduction of a sand pit to the enclosure may allow the rabbit to dig without damaging the garden. Initially, the sand pit should be introduced while the animals are living on the concrete to enable the owner to find the appropriate substrate and allow time for the rabbit to create an association. The sand pit should be deep enough for the rabbit to dig to a depth equivalent to its height and wide enough for the rabbit to be able to turn around.

The other issue is the choice of a guinea pig as a companion. With the female rabbit not having been neutered, there is a possibility that it might start to display sexual behaviour towards the guinea pig, or vice versa. The danger is that either individual could use aggression to ward off these advances and, given the size difference, the outcome may not be pleasant. Many people keep a guinea pig and a rabbit together but it is worth first considering the sexual status of both individuals, the ability of either animal to retreat from the other and the temperament of each animal, in addition to ensuring that the environment is appropriately sized.

## CASE 18

On routine surgical exposure of the abdomen in rabbits, what anatomical structures are located immediately below the incision site and should therefore be carefully avoided (18)? Care should be taken when entering the abdominal cavity in the rabbit because the abdominal musculature is thin and overzealous surgical technique could result in iatrogenic damage to the underlying soft tissue structures. These include the small intestines, the very large thin-walled caecum situated on the right side of the abdomen and the bladder caudally. Grasping the body wall with forceps and elevating it away from underlying structures prior to making an incision will help avoid iatrogenic damage.

## CASE 19

1 **Given the species and geographic location, what is your main differential?** Based on the time frame of late summer and the geographic location in the South Central USA, one should be suspicious of tularaemia. Other differentials for this acute, fatal neurological presentation in a wild rabbit include rabies virus, neural larval migrans of *Baylisascaris procyonis* or trauma. The aetiological agent of tularaemia is *Francisella tularensis*, an aerobic non-motile, Gram-negative, pleomorphic, non-capsulated, bipolar rod or coccobacillus. The pathogenesis of disease is poorly understood but may involve an endotoxin. *F. tularensis* causes an acute fatal septicaemia; necropsy findings include pulmonary congestion and consolidation, multiple small white hepatic foci and subpleural petechial haemorrhage. Granulomatous lesions within multiple organs and lymph nodes may be present. Impression stains of lesions will reveal intra- and extracellular small Gram-negative coccobacilli.

2 **What is your next step?** Tularaemia is a reportable disease in the USA, so the appropriate local agriculture and public health departments should be contacted immediately. Because humans are highly susceptible to tularaemia via contact with infected animals, employee exposure to this animal should be restricted; gloves and masks should be worn by anyone handling the carcass. Remains should be sent to an adequate biohazard facility for necropsy as directed by the State department of agriculture.

3 **How would you advise the man who brought the rabbit in?** The man who brought the rabbit in should be notified of your suspicion of potential tularaemia. Up to 90% of human cases of tularaemia have been linked to wild lagomorph exposure. Humans may also be exposed via ingestion of contaminated water or partially cooked meat, inhalation of faecal droplets (e.g. during lawn mowing in endemic areas) or bites from infected blood-sucking arthropods such as *Dermacenter variablis*, *D. andersonnii*, *Amblyomma americanum* or *Chrisops discalis*. The most common presentation of tularaemia in humans is the ulceroglandular form. The man who found the rabbit should seek advice from his personal physician as soon as possible.

## CASE 20

**What anaesthetic circuit and associated equipment is suitable for gaseous anaesthesia in rabbits (20)?** Adult rabbit bodyweight varies from 500 g to 10 kg; therefore, equipment designed for cats and small dogs is usually suitable. The volume of dead space must be low; therefore, an Ayre's T-piece or unmodified Bain's circuit is most suitable. The tidal volume of an anaesthetized rabbit can be as low as 5–10 ml/kg, so low dead space connectors can be used for small patients less than 2 kg. Connectors used in human paediatric anaesthesia may be used. In an intubated rabbit, assisted ventilation can be achieved either manually using a reservoir bag on the end of a T-piece or unmodified Bain's circuit, or by using a mechanical ventilator capable of delivering low tidal volumes. In-line devices may be used to humidify and warm inspired gases, but these will contribute to dead space.

## CASE 21

**1 What are the lesion(s) observed in the photograph (21) taken at postmortem examination?** The photograph shows the heart, which is pale and has hypertrophy of the ventricles. There is a thrombus firmly attached to the left atrial wall.

**2 What is the most likely cause of the postmortem changes in this animal?** The most likely cause of the observed postmortem changes is idiopathic hypertrophic cardiomyopathy. Other types of heart disease include other cardiomyopathies (dilated and secondary to chronic stress), myocarditis (secondary to *Encephalitozoon cuniculi*, *Salmonella* spp. or coronavirus infection), myocardial fibrosis, pericarditis (secondary to *Pasteurella multocida* or *Staphylococcus* spp. infection), valvular disease (mitral and tricuspid insufficiencies and endocarditis) and congenital defects (atrial and ventricular septal defects and haemocyst).

## CASE 22

**1 What lesion is shown in the lateral radiograph of the lumbar spine (22)?** A fracture of the 6th lumbar vertebra.

**2 How would you determine a prognosis, and what emergency treatment would you consider?** The prognosis depends on the degree of compromise to the spinal cord. In the rabbit the spinal cord extends the length of the spinal column, so that in this case there is likely to be upper motor neuron damage with some lower motor neuron involvement as well. This should be assessed by standard neurological tests such as anal sphincter tone, cutaneous skin sensation, bladder control, hindlimb reflexes and pain sensation. Absence of deep pain sensation in the rabbit carries a poor prognosis; however, because they conceal signs of pain, this test is not always reliable in rabbits. Withdrawal of the hindlimbs can be a local reflex and may still occur with a transected spinal cord. If the spinal cord is transected, the prognosis is poor and euthanasia may be indicated. If sensation is demonstrable, stabilization of the spine might allow recovery. Internal fixation may have a poor prognosis, as the bone density of the vertebrae is often reduced and secure anchoring of implants may not be feasible. There are no reports of a successful technique for repairing spinal fractures in rabbits, but spinal fusion has been reported in laboratory rabbits. Osteoporosis may result from lack of exercise in caged rabbits and this increases the risk of spinal fractures when excessive stresses are involved, such as struggling when handled incorrectly. Cart and trolley systems have been used in paraplegic rabbits to support the hindlimbs in cases where owners are prepared to nurse the animal sufficiently, but any associated welfare implications must be thoroughly assessed. Pressure sores are common and faecal and urinary incontinence will need to be managed. Where there is a chance that normal neurological function will return, supportive care with cage rest should be commenced. In acute cases, shock doses of i/v methylprednisolone may be administered, although the efficacy of this treatment remains controversial. The bladder may need regular manual expression to avoid urine retention problems. Long-term analgesia and anti-inflammatory drugs are also indicated. Euthanasia should be considered.

## CASE 23

**What advice would you give about managing this situation?** Firstly, both rabbits should be examined to ensure that neither is in pain, as this can lead to random aggression and/or unpredictable behaviour.

It is possible that the owner's interpretation of 'happily moving from one cage to another' is not correct. Rabbits can be very territorial and does can be quite aggressive if another rabbit enters their territory; for example, when mating rabbits, a breeder has to ensure that the doe is placed in the buck's hutch. In addition to territorial aggression, there are other motivations to be considered. There may have been aggression over a resource such as a food bowl or proximity to the owner (if the rabbits are attached to her). Rabbits can display aggression towards a conspecific if they are frightened by environmental stimuli. This is a displaced behaviour.

It is important that the owner tries to reintroduce the rabbits, assuming the injury to the male rabbit will not affect his confidence or leave him visually impaired. If either rabbit has not been neutered, then it is helpful to perform the operation at this point.

Initially, the owner should move the indoor cages close together so that the rabbits are in the same room but can have only visual access. She should have a better idea of the prognosis for this problem at this point. All being well, the rabbits should ignore each other or sleep alongside each other. With time and success each rabbit can be let out of the cage alternately. If there is any mutual grooming (through the bars of the cage), that is a sign of acceptance.

In the meantime the owner should be advised to prepare a neutral environment for the rabbits to meet in – this is usually a room in the house that they have not been in before. The owner should ensure that the room has lots of areas for the rabbits to retreat to and several food sources.

Assuming that this and subsequent meetings are successful, the owner should be prepared to purchase a large indoor cage that both rabbits can share, and move them back to their original environment.

## CASE 24

**1 Name the vessels indicated in 24.** (1) Intermediate ramus of the caudal auricular artery; (2) caudal auricular vein, commonly referred to as the marginal ear vein.

**2 Why should vessel 1 be used with care for blood sampling?** As this is an artery, its use for blood sampling or drug administration carries a risk of haematoma or thrombosis development. This can lead to sloughing of the associated skin, necrosis of part of the cartilage or even loss of part of the pinna in severe cases, due to an avascular necrosis. However, many clinicians and laboratory technicians do use this artery routinely for blood sampling or blood gas analysis during anaesthetic monitoring without problems. Careful technique and the application of sustained pressure after sampling should be employed.

## CASE 25

**1 Why is the rabbit likely to be inappetant?** Most rabbits are already displaying clinical signs of inappetance +/– secondary gastrointestinal stasis at the time of diagnosis of dental disease, particularly if oral trauma is present. This can largely be attributed to pain and can take time to resolve post dental procedure. Furthermore, the secondary effects of a general anaesthetic on gastrointestinal motility can result in the rabbit requiring a number of days of assisted syringe feeding, until normal voluntary dietary intake resumes. These effects can be minimized by appropriate pre-anaesthetic stabilization of the patient with fluid therapy, analgesia, prokinetic drugs and assisted feeding.

**2 What postoperative medication would be appropriate for this case?** Analgesia is essential to encourage eating and acceptance of a more fibrous diet as soon as possible after the procedure. Sources of pain include ulceration caused by spurs, exposure of sensitive dentine and stretching of masticatory muscles. Antibiosis is required in the presence of ulceration or periodontal/periapical infection. Gastrointestinal motility stimulants help prevent ileus, especially in a previously anorexic patient, as does syringe feeding of a critical-care herbivore diet. The latter also helps to maintain a positive energy and fluid balance, and correct previous nutritional deficiencies. Appropriate fluid therapy should also be continued as required in the postoperative period.

**3 What is the likely prognosis in this case?** In early mild cases, dentistry and an improved diet may be curative, though this situation is rare. However, changes in shape, position and direction of growth of teeth are permanent and so malocclusion will recur, requiring further repeated dentistry procedures. The majority of dental disease cases present with moderate to advanced clinical signs, therefore long-term management of these cases is more realistic to achieve than a cure. In cases of severe dental disease, euthanasia on welfare grounds should be a consideration, based on clinical findings, radiography and CT imaging techniques. Cases should be discussed carefully with the owner at the outset to ensure that a realistic treatment plan is achieved.

## CASE 26

**1 What are your differential diagnoses?** Careful examination is always important to differentiate exophthalmos from globe enlargement (buphthalmos). If confirmed to be exophthalmos, differentials include: retrobulbar abscess (often unilateral and related to dental disease), retrobulbar neoplasia, idiopathic retrobulbar adenitis or congestion of the retrobulbar venous sinuses (e.g. due to a mediastinal mass compressing the anterior vena cava). Mediastinal masses such as thymomas are the most common cause of bilateral exophthalmos and in these cases eyes can usually be easily retropulsed, unlike in cases with retrobulbar abscesses or neoplasia where there is often marked resistance.

**2 What diagnostics would you recommend to confirm your diagnosis?** Skull and thoracic radiography is recommended to determine if exophthalmos is due to a retrobulbar or mediastinal lesion. In the case of a mediastinal mass, a rounded soft tissue opacity is generally visible cranial to the heart. A CT scan will provide more detailed information if available or alternatively ocular ultrasound may be used to identify a retrobulbar mass. If a mediastinal mass is identified, an ultrasound-guided fine-needle aspirate of the mass will help differentiate between thymoma and thymic lymphoma.

## CASE 27

1 **What opioid analgesics are commonly used in rabbits, and what is their duration of action?**

| Opioid | Dose (mg/kg) | Method | Duration of action (hours) |
|---|---|---|---|
| Buprenorphine | 0.05–0.1 | s/c, i/v | 6–12 |
| Butorphanol | 0.1–0.5 | s/c, i/v | 2–4 |
| Morphine | 2–5 | s/c | 2–4 |
| Pethidine (meperidine) | 5–10 | s/c | 2–4 |
| Nalbuphine | 1–2 | i/v | 2–4 |

2 **What can they be used for in addition to analgesia?** Buprenorphine and butorphanol can be used to reverse the action of fentanyl (a component of the licensed product fentanyl/fluanisone) while maintaining some analgesia.

3 **What are the undesirable side effects of opioids?** Potential side effects are respiratory depression and reduced gut motility. In practice the risks associated with these side effects are of minimal significance in the rabbit and they are greatly outweighed by the benefits of providing good analgesia. For example, the effects of pain itself in causing reduced gut motility are likely to be far more of a risk than that of an opioid.

## CASE 28

1 **What word best describes this condition?** Myiasis, defined as the infestation of living animals with dipteran fly larvae. The larva embedded in the neck of this rabbit is most likely a *Cuterebra* spp. (order Diptera, family Cuterebridae), also called the rabbit botfly. Adult *Cuterebra* flies are large and do not bite or suck blood. The females lay eggs around the openings of animal nests and burrows or on plants and stones in these areas. The larvae enter the host through the mouth or nares during grooming, or through open wounds. The larvae then migrate to subcutaneous locations along the dorsum, axillary, inguinal and ventral cervical areas, where they pupate and form a breathing hole to the surface. For the most part, other than local pain and inflammation, rabbits are systemically unaffected by *Cuterebra* infestation. However, some rabbits can present for lameness, or are weak, anorectic and/or dehydrated. Larvae can be up to 25 × 10 mm (1 × 0.4 inches) in size and have black cuticular spines, which give them their characteristic dark appearance.

**2 Describe your treatment and prevention plan.** First, a thorough physical examination should be conducted to ensure that no more larvae are present on the rabbit. Mild sedation or general anaesthesia may be required for larval removal. After preparing the area for surgery, the air hole should be gently expanded with haemostat tips. The larva should then be pulled through the widened opening. There are anecdotal reports of larval rupture causing anaphylaxis in the host, so care must be taken to remove the larva in one piece. After larval removal, the area should be thoroughly flushed with sterile saline and debrided as needed. Oral analgesics and antibiotics should be prescribed. If the swelling does not resolve or if it worsens, surgical excision of the affected tissues may be necessary. The owner should be advised that the best prevention is to limit exposure of the rabbit to flies, either by keeping the rabbit indoors during the fly season or installing a protective screen over the hutch.

## CASE 29

**1 What are the dental formulas (deciduous and permanent) of the rabbit (29)?**
Deciduous: I 2/1  C 0/0  P 3/2  M 0/0 = 16 (shed just before or just after birth)
Permanent: I 2/1  C 0/0  P 3/2  M 3/3 = 28

**2 Describe the normal dental anatomy and function.** The occlusal surface of the larger first incisors is chisel-like in lateral profile (about 45° upper, 30° lower) by virtue of the differential distribution of enamel on the labial and lingual sides. The smaller second upper incisor, usually known as the 'peg tooth' and a characteristic of lagomorphs, is located just caudal to the first, such that the tips of the lower incisors come to rest just between the two. Unlike most rodents, the incisor enamel is non-pigmented. There is then a gap (the diastema) between the incisors and the premolars. The latter are of similar morphology to the molars and so together they are often referred to as the 'cheek' or 'molariform' teeth. These possess transverse ridges and the plane of the occlusal surface is approximately 10° to the horizontal.

Rabbits are anisognathous, meaning that the distance between the left and right upper cheek tooth arcades is greater than that of the lower cheek teeth so the buccal edge of the upper arcade just occludes with the lingual edge of the lower arcade. The temporomandibular articulation is dorsal to the longitudinal occlusal. The mobile lips and rostral tongue prehend the vegetation, which is cropped by the vertical, scissor-like action of the incisors. However, the gnawing function of the incisors is performed by a rostrocaudal movement of the mandible. The food material is then moved caudally by the tongue and ground by the lateral movement of the mandibular cheek teeth. A consequence of the anisognathism is that mastication takes place on alternate sides, but in equal measure, and utilizing the entire width of the occlusal surface.

## CASE 30

**1 What is the lesion?** Prolapse of the deep gland of the nictitating membrane causing swelling and protrusion of the third eyelid. Prolapse is associated with gland hyperplasia.

**2 How would you treat this case?** The gland may be surgically replaced using a similar technique to that described in the dog. This is the preferred technique, since it preserves the gland's secretory function; however, this technique may not be possible due to the increased size of the gland and, in this instance, surgical excision would be the preferred option. This should be performed with great care as the base of the gland is close to the orbital sinus, with the consequent risk of significant haemorrhage. The prognosis is good in cases where the gland is surgically replaced. Topical antibiotic ophthalmic ointment should be applied to the eye for five days post surgery.

## CASE 31

**1 Identify the indicated cell on the rapid Romanovsky-type (Rapid-Diff) stained blood smear shown (31).** A neutrophil, also referred to by some authors as a rabbit heterophil.

**2 Is the morphology normal, and, if not, why?** The morphology is normal. The neutrophil is a granulocyte, and eosinophilic cytoplasmic granules are normally visible on smears. Neutrophils need to be differentiated from eosinophils, which in the rabbit are bigger cells, with larger round eosinophilic granules. These may obscure the cell nucleus. In the majority of cases, neutrophils will be the most numerous granulocytic cell in a rabbit blood smear.

## CASE 32

**1 What is the most likely cause of this rabbit's clinical signs?** Based on the history of a raccoon bite a month ago and the clinical signs, this rabbit is highly likely to have the raccoon variant of the rabies virus. The rabies virus is a rhabdovirus transmitted by saliva carrying the virus into the tissues via a bite from an infected animal. It causes an acute encephalomyelitis that is most common in carnivorous mammals and insectivorous bats. It has been theorized that rabies is less common in rabbits and other small rodents, as they are less likely to survive an animal attack. Rabbits most commonly develop the paralytic form of the disease. Clinical signs in experimentally infected rabbits include anorexia, hyperthermia and restlessness, progressing to weight loss and the development of neurological signs, such as those displayed by this rabbit, and ascending paralysis. Because antemortem testing lacks sensitivity, the appropriate next step in this case is to euthanase the rabbit and submit its head to the appropriate testing laboratory as determined by State laws for rabies testing. Direct immunofluorescent antibody testing is performed on brain tissues, particularly the hippocampus, medulla oblongata and cerebellum.

**2 Should you do anything with the asymptomatic rabbit that also lives in the hutch?** If the results from rabies testing on this rabbit's brain come back positive, the local health department may require that the asymptomatic rabbit is also euthanased and its brain sent for testing.

## CASE 33

**1 Hepatic coccidiosis increases the body's requirement for which two vitamins?** Liver disease caused by *Eimeria stiedae* can interfere with the metabolism of the fat-soluble vitamins A and E.

**2 What clinical signs may be observed in rabbits with deficiencies of these two vitamins?** In breeding rabbits a dietary deficiency of vitamins A and/or E may be associated with problems such as infertility, embryonic/fetal resorption, abortion, stillbirth and neonatal death. In addition, suboptimal vitamin A levels have resulted in hydrocephalus and cerebellar malformation in newborns and stunted growth rates and weight loss in juvenile rabbits. In adults, ocular lesions ranging from keratitis, iridocyclitis and hypopyon through to permanent blindness have been associated with vitamin A deficiency. Other manifestations include enteritis and neurological abnormalities.

As well as the consequences for fertility and breeding success, vitamin E deficiency in rabbits may result in muscular dystrophy and hindlimb weakness, as it does in other species.

## CASE 34

**1 What abnormalities can be seen?** The surgical skin wounds are intact. There is some bilateral scrotal swelling present, more obvious in the left scrotum.

**2 What are the differential diagnoses, and what further investigative procedures should be carried out?** Postoperative bruising/haemorrhage; infection; herniation of abdominal contents via the inguinal canal. A full history should be taken and the rabbit examined to assess whether it is systemically unwell and if any GI problems are present. Ultrasonographic examination of the affected area should help rule out the presence of abdominal contents. If the swellings are warm and painful, a fine-needle aspirate may be used to check for infection. Any aspirate should be examined cytologically and cultured. However, the veterinary surgeon should be aware that the swellings may contain intestines, and so exploratory surgery and appropriate repair may be indicated. In this case the swellings were due to postoperative bruising, and the patient responded to a 5-day course of NSAID therapy. Analgesia is important postoperatively to reduce discomfort and also reduce the risk of self-trauma leading to wound dehiscence.

## CASE 35

**1 Give one advantage and one disadvantage of each type of food over the other.**
Extruded pellets, which are produced by steam heating ground raw ingredients, are manufactured in various sizes and shapes. They have the advantage of being homogeneous (i.e. eliminating the possibility of selective eating) and the manufacturing process essentially sterilizes the ingredients. They provide a consistent ration supplemented with vitamins and minerals that can, when fed in limited amounts, act as a balancer for hay, grass and other fresh items (that may be of variable nutritional value). However, these pellets do not provide high quantities of non-digestible fibre and are often less appealing to owners aesthetically.

Mixed rations ('mueslis') vary in their composition depending on the source. Most contain a variety of cereals and legumes mixed with dried vegetables and highly coloured biscuits or pellets, and they are therefore often deemed more visually appealing to the owner. However, the majority of these constituents are low in fibre and high in starch. Mixed rations encourage selective feeding and therefore are often associated with an unbalanced intake of nutrients. Some of these products are sold loose in pet stores, with no labelling information provided. Some may contain chunks of locust bean, which have been implicated in cases of gastrointestinal obstructions. Both types of food are popular as they are highly palatable, convenient and readily available. However, dietary studies have shown that mixed ration (muesli-type) diets are associated with the development of obesity, dental disease, reduced gastrointestinal motility and abnormal behaviours in rabbits.

**2 Is either of these foods suitable as a complete *ad libitum* diet for adult or geriatric pet rabbits?** Although some concentrates are marketed as complete diets, this claim and their formulation is based on the nutritional requirements of commercially farmed rabbits, which live short lives. In non-breeding adult and geriatric pet rabbits, concentrates should only be used in limited amounts as complementary feedstuffs, with the bulk of the diet being provided by good quality hay and grasses. Recent dietary studies in pet rabbits have indicated that mixed muesli-type rations are not recommended, and extruded nuggets or pellets with fibre levels >18% are preferred.

**3 How should these foods be stored?** The optimum storage conditions for commercial feeds are a cool (15 °C [59 °F]), dry, vermin-proof place and they should be fed within 90 days of the milling date. Owners should be discouraged from purchasing concentrate feeds in large quantities for small numbers of rabbits, as food more than 6 months old may have a compromised nutritional quality due to degradation of vitamin content, especially if stored at high temperatures.

## CASE 36

An encapsulated abscess is shown, following its surgical removal from the subcutaneous tissue on the lateral cervical neck of a rabbit (36). **Describe how you would obtain a sample for bacterial culture in this case.** Attempts at obtaining a fine needle aspirate of a rabbit abscess are usually unsuccessful, since rabbit pus is thick and caseous. The material at the centre of the abscess is likely to be sterile and best culture results are obtained by culturing the abscess wall or capsule. Sections of tissue give the best culture results, rather than capsular swabs. It is important to culture for both aerobic and anaerobic bacteria, since it is common to find that anaerobic bacteria are involved, particularly in dental abscesses.

## CASE 37

**What emergency procedures should you carry out in an anaesthetized rabbit in which respiratory arrest has occurred (37)?** Respiratory arrest must be dealt with immediately, as cardiac arrest due to hypoxia can rapidly ensue. If the rabbit is intubated or has a tight-fitting laryngeal mask in place, assisted breathing should be instituted by intermittently squeezing the reservoir bag of a T-piece or Bain's circuit. Any volatile agent should be switched off and 100% oxygen used to ventilate the animal. Reversal agents to injectable anaesthetics (e.g. atipamezole or naloxone) should be given if appropriate. The respiratory stimulant doxapram can be administered intravenously (2–5 mg/kg) if venous access is available, sublingually, or intralingually (i/m). If the rabbit is not intubated, oxygen by face mask should be given. The rabbit can be rocked (held in dorsal recumbency and the head and rear end elevated and dropped alternately in a 'see-saw' action) to move the diaphragm in and out. Breathing movements in the rabbit are mainly diaphragmatic and this is an effective way of ventilating the animal. Attempts to ventilate using a face mask invariably result in inflation of the stomach, not the lungs. This can create further problems as the inflated stomach puts pressure on the diaphragm, and the inability of rabbits to eructate will result in gastric tympany.

## CASE 38

**1 What is the condition shown?** This is a blepharitis, most likely to be bacterial in aetiology. Another differential diagnosis would be myxomatosis, but this is less likely due to the unilateral change and acute onset.

**2 What diagnostic tests would you perform in this case, and how would you treat the patient while waiting for results?** Samples for microbiological investigation should be taken by expressing the contents of the meibomian glands in the eyelid margins. Swabbing the contents of the conjunctival sac is more likely to reveal a mixed bacterial growth, with contaminating microbes of minimal significance.

This is an infection of the eyelid as opposed to the conjunctiva and should be treated with systemic antibiotics, rather than just topical antibiosis. The preferred medication is a suitable systemic broad-spectrum antibiotic until results of culture and sensitivity determine a more specific drug. Typical culture results would indicate *Staphylococcus* spp., but other infections may be demonstrated.

## CASE 39

**1 What immediate treatment would you consider?** Immediate treatment should consist of oxygen therapy (in a cage to minimize stress). Severely distressed patients may be sedated with midazolam (1 mg/kg i/m).

**2 What are the differential diagnoses for this rabbit?** Traumatic tracheitis as a result of endotracheal intubation is the most likely diagnosis in a rabbit with this history and clinical signs. Other differential diagnoses include foreign body inhalation, severe tracheitis secondary to irritants (ammonia, smoke), and extraluminal abscess.

**3 How would you confirm your diagnosis?** Further investigation will be limited by the stability and size of the patient. General anaesthesia and tracheoscopy are required to visualize the trachea. Lateral cervical and thoracic radiographs should be evaluated for abnormalities to rule out other causes of stridor and dyspnoea. In this case, however, the owner elected for euthanasia. Severe necrotizing tracheitis and submucosal oedema were found on postmortem examination.

## CASE 40

**What factors should be considered when deciding the route of administration of an antibiotic drug to a pet rabbit (40)?** The aim is to obtain an effective concentration of the antibiotic at the infection site for the duration it takes to kill the bacteria. Certain oral antibiotic preparations may induce enteritis and diarrhoea in rabbits due to disturbance of the normal hindgut microflora (caecal dysbiosis) and overgrowth of potential toxin-forming pathogens such as *Clostridia* spp., so great care should be taken when choosing which antibiotic to use. Antibiotics such as cephalosporins, many penicillins, clindamycin, erythromycin and lincomycin will induce enteritis if given orally, but they may be safe if given parenterally. Ampicillin, amoxycillin and amoxycillin-clavulanic should not be given to rabbits by any route, as there is a high risk of fatal acid enterotoxaemia associated with these drugs. Some oral preparations may be bitter tasting (e.g. fluoroquinolones) and this may cause difficulties in administration. If a rabbit has intestinal ileus, an oral preparation may not be well absorbed from the intestine and the parenteral route may be preferable. Some antibiotics cause localized tissue reactions when given by s/c or i/m injection (e.g. enrofloxacin). Which of these two routes is chosen will depend on the volume of fluid to be injected and the required absorption rate. In a debilitated rabbit s/c injections may not be as rapidly absorbed as i/m ones. Obese rabbits may have large subcutaneous fat deposits, which will have poor drug absorption. Intravenous antibiotic administration is not always practical, except perhaps in a hospitalized animal with placement of an indwelling catheter. Administration of antibiotics via the drinking water is not recommended, since this relies on the animal drinking sufficient amounts of water to reach therapeutic doses. The water often becomes less palatable. Where infection occurs at inaccessible sites, antibiotics may be injected directly into the site or administered via implantation of antibiotic-impregnated beads to obtain high drug concentrations at the site of infection. Care should be taken when prescribing topical antibiotic preparations, as these may be ingested following grooming and can lead to enteritis.

## CASE 41

**1 Give four examples of injectable balanced anaesthetic regimes suitable for surgical procedures.** Regimes commonly used include:
- fentanyl/fluanisone + diazepam or midazolam (0.2–0.5 ml/kg + 0.5–2.0 mg/kg, i/m or s/c)
- ketamine/medetomidine (15 mg/kg + 0.25 mg/kg, s/c)
- ketamine/medetomidine/butorphanol (15 mg/kg + 0.25 mg/kg + 0.4 mg/kg, i/m or s/c)
- ketamine/xylazine (35 mg/kg + 5 mg/kg, i/m or s/c)
- ketamine/xylazine/butorphanol (35 mg/kg + 5 mg/kg + 0.4 mg/kg, i/m or s/c)
- ketamine/xylazine/acepromazine (35 mg/kg + 5 mg/kg + 1 mg/kg, i/m or s/c)
- ketamine/diazepam (25 mg/kg + 5 mg/kg, i/m or s/c)
- ketamine/acepromazine (50 mg/kg + 1 mg/kg, i/m or s/c).

(NB: For all these regimes, 100% oxygen should be administered by mask or via endotracheal tube.)

**2 Are any injectable anaesthetics licensed for use in the rabbit in the UK?** Only fentanyl/fluanisone is licensed in the UK.

## CASE 42

**1 If only 0.5 ml of blood is sampled from an 800 g Netherland Dwarf rabbit (42), which anticoagulant should be selected to allow both haematology and serum biochemistry to be performed on the same sample?** Storing the blood sample in heparin will allow a laboratory to perform haematology and most biochemistry on the sample. If sufficient blood can be taken, it is preferable to submit an ethylenediamine tetra-acetic acid (EDTA) sample for haematology and a heparin sample for biochemistry. Heparin is more advantageous than plain serum tube samples, as small samples yield a larger volume of plasma than serum on centrifugation, and the sample is less likely to need dilution to run a panel of biochemistry tests.

**2 What is the disadvantage of selecting this anticoagulant for haematology?** While preventing coagulation, heparin may cause clumping of leukocytes, and this can give a lower leukocyte count than EDTA samples. This is more obviously seen when counts are performed manually in a haemocytometer. A fresh blood smear should always be examined or submitted to the external laboratory, as heparin alters the staining characteristics of the leukocytes.

**3 Why is it inadvisable to flush the sampling syringe with heparin or heparin–saline before blood sampling?** Preflushing a syringe with heparin–saline when sampling small rabbits, or using the marginal ear vein, can cause significant dilution artefacts. The residual volume of most 1 ml or 2 ml syringes (the hub and needle space) is approximately 0.05–0.08 ml, with the exception of insulin syringes, where this may be less than 0.02 ml. In a 0.5 ml blood sample this can cause a >10% error in haematology and biochemistry parameters. This will make marginally abnormal and normal haematology and biochemistry parameters difficult to interpret, and it may lead to an erroneous diagnosis being made. Heparin may also cause clumping of leukocytes, affecting the leukocyte count. As heparin changes the staining characteristics of the leukocytes, a fresh blood smear is recommended for performing the differential white cell count.

## CASE 43

**1 What temperature should the incubator be set at initially and as the rabbit recovers further?** A temperature of approximately 35 °C is appropriate initially. Rabbits will remain susceptible to hypothermia until normal activity is regained. The temperature can be dropped to 26–28 °C as the rabbit regains consciousness. Only when the rabbit is fully recovered should it be returned to comfortable room temperature (21–22 °C).

**2 List the other components of supportive care that the rabbit should receive in the postoperative period.** Analgesia; fluid therapy if required (i/v, s/c; warmed); motility stimulants to prevent ileus (e.g. metoclopramide, cisapride); transfer to a cage once recovered, with plentiful good quality hay and greens to encourage eating as soon as possible; assisted feeding with a high-fibre paste if not eating voluntarily within 4–6 hours; quiet darkened area with hidebox away from predator species.

## CASE 44

**1 What are your differential diagnoses?** Differential diagnoses are *Treponema paraluis cuniculi*, myxoma virus infection, and other bacterial or fungal infection, for example with *Staphylococcus aureus*. *Treponema* infection (rabbit syphilis) manifests as redness and oedema of the external genitalia, followed by vesicles and scabs. Lesions can also be found on the head, around the muzzle, and on the forelimbs, from autoinoculation. Myxomatosis in rabbits causes swelling of the mucocutaneous junctions of the anogenital region, as well as swelling of the head, ears and eyelids. Bacterial or fungal infection with other agents such as *S. aureus* is less common but could cause anogenital swelling.

**2 What further diagnostic tests would you perform?** Diagnosis of rabbit syphilis involves identification of the organism by dark-field microscopy of scrapings, histology using silver dye, polymerase chain reaction (PCR), or serology. Bacterial and fungal culture may also be indicated. Skin biopsies should be taken to differentiate between *Treponema* and myxomatosis infections in the absence of other clinical signs.

## CASE 45

**Describe how you would perform an enucleation in a rabbit (45a, b). How does this surgical procedure differ in the rabbit compared with enucleation in cats and dogs?** The surgical procedure of enucleation is similar to that in other small animals. A transconjunctival technique is used, with careful dissection along the globe, to avoid trauma to the orbital sinus. Rabbits have a large ophthalmic venous sinus. If haemorrhage occurs, it is often significant; however, it can usually be controlled with pressure. Once freed, a haemostatic clip should be applied to the optic nerve and blood vessels prior to enucleation (45c). If infection is present, the orbit should be lavaged copiously with warm saline and appropriate antibiosis administered.

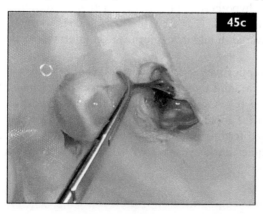

Placement of AIPMMA beads into the surgical site may be indicated in cases with retrobulbar abscess formation; also administration of long-term systemic procaine penicillin following surgery. Postoperative drains are rarely useful and are not well tolerated. The only differences with this procedure in rabbits compared with that in dogs and cats are the large venous sinuses surrounding the muscle cone and the Harderian gland posterior to the globe, which should be avoided and may act as a source of considerable haemorrhage. Analgesia (e.g. buprenorphine [0.05 mg/kg s/c q6–8h]) should be continued in the postoperative period to reduce the likelihood of self-trauma to the surgical site.

## CASE 46

**1 What are the indications for the use of an antimuscarinic (parasympatholytic) agent in rabbit anaesthetic protocols?** Antimuscarinic agents are used preoperatively to decrease oral and bronchial secretions and to inhibit vagal efferent activity and bradycardia. They may also be used with anticholinesterase drugs such as neostigmine during the antagonism of neuromuscular blockade. Routine use for pre-anaesthetic medication is controversial and some anaesthetists reserve their use for only when problems of excessive secretion or bradycardia occur.

**2 What agent is most suitable in this species and why?** Glycopyrronium bromide. The alternative drug, atropine, may only be short-acting, as a large proportion of rabbits are believed to have serum atropinesterase. Glycopyrronium is longer-acting than atropine and, being a quaternary ammonium compound, does not readily cross the blood–brain barrier or placental barrier, thus reducing the risk of possible adverse effects if overdosed.

**3 What commonly used drug in rabbits can be antagonized by antimuscarinics?** Metoclopramide.

## CASE 47

**1 What are the differential diagnoses in this case?** Retrobulbar space-occupying lesion, such as an abscess (possibly associated with tooth root overgrowth), neoplasia (e.g. lymphoma) or tapeworm cyst (*T. serialis*); orbital cellulitis – usually associated with dental disease; increased intraocular pressure such as glaucoma, infection, haemorrhage or neoplasia. Exophthalmos may also occur in rabbits with an intrathoracic mass (e.g. thymoma, mediastinal lymphoma), and following long-term external jugular catheter placement, but this is usually bilateral due to reduced venous return to the heart.

**2 What further investigative procedures would you perform?** Ophthalmoscopy may detect ocular infiltrates. Intraocular pressure measurements will be elevated in glaucoma. Oral examination and radiography of the skull is indicated to rule out underlying dental disease. Ultrasonography of the orbit may demonstrate an abscess, and needle aspiration may be used to sample the contents. Aspirates are likely to be purulent material associated with *Pasteurella multocida* or other bacterial infection. Imaging using computed tomography (CT) is very useful for visualising any mass and its relation to bony structures, and for detection of dental disease.

## CASE 48

**1 What cestode infections occur in rabbits, and how do they present?** The rabbit is the intermediate host for *Taenia pisiformis* and *T. serialis*. The dog is the definitive host; rabbits, however, can become infected if eating grass contaminated by infected dog and wild fox faeces. The intermediate stages can be found in rabbits,

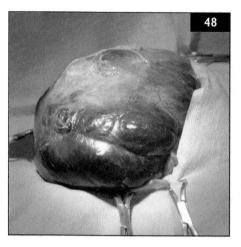

with cysticerci in the mesentery and liver and coenuri in the muscle and connective tissue. The latter may present as large subcutaneous fluid filled cysts (**48**).

**2 What is the treatment of choice for cestode infection in rabbits?** Praziquantel (6 mg/kg s/c, repeated 10 days later) has been used to treat tapeworm infection in pet rabbits. Surgical removal of subcutaneous cysts may be achieved, or percutaneous drainage in addition to treatment with praziquantel.

## CASE 49

**Explain the terms diphyodont, heterodont and aradicular hypsodont, which describe the dental anatomy and physiology of the rabbit, and comment on the clinical significance of aradicular hypsodont.** Diphydont – There are two sets of teeth during the life of the rabbit; the deciduous or primary teeth are shed *in utero*.

Heterodont – The dentition consists of teeth of different anatomical types. The term 'hypsodont' refers to teeth in which the crown length is greater than that of the root, although the majority of it remains below the gum level and progressively erupts as the exposed crown is worn down. All the teeth of lagomorphs and hystricomorphs (guinea pigs and chinchillas) and the incisors of myomorphs (rats, mice, gerbils and hamsters) are aradicular hypsodont, characterized by the absence of a true root (aradicular), and are often misleadingly called 'open-rooted'. The germinal tissue at the tooth apex (relatively lucent areas on the lateral radiograph of the normal skull shown [49]) continuously produces new crown, which erupts as the occlusal surface is worn away during mastication of abrasive food material. The parts of the tooth are therefore properly referred to as 'reserve crown' (that which is embedded in alveolar bone) and 'exposed crown', rather than crown and root. The mandibular teeth grow and erupt faster than those of the maxilla. One study ascertained a rate of approximately 13 cm (5.2 inches) per year for the upper incisors and 20 cm (8 inches) per year for the lower. This process continues at a rate that ensures a constant exposed crown length, in equilibrium with the rate of attrition caused by tooth-on-tooth wear and the rabbit's natural diet of grass and other fibrous herbage. If the rate of wear is reduced, either due to

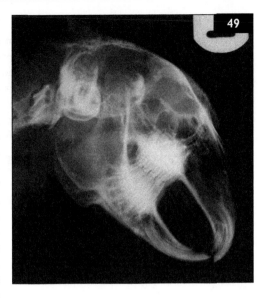

malocclusion or inappropriate food, the tooth will elongate abnormally. The rate of growth and attrition varies between individuals and is influenced by factors such as pregnancy, age and diet.

## CASE 50

**1 What are the advantages of inducing anaesthesia prior to euthanasia in a pet rabbit?** This drug combination is particularly useful in reducing stress in fractious or aggressive animals. Operator stress is reduced, since administration of the euthanasia agent is easier in an immobile animal, especially when owners are present. Involuntary movements or muscle spasms are less likely to occur when using a pre-euthanasia anaesthetic combination.

**2 What are the advantages of using this particular anaesthetic combination?** A relatively small volume may be injected subcutaneously. This combination results in a smooth but relatively rapid onset of anaesthesia (within 20–30 minutes). The combination provides good analgesia.

**3 What are the disadvantages of using this particular anaesthetic combination?** This combination produces moderate peripheral vasoconstriction, making i/v catheter placement or peripheral venepuncture more difficult. The owner should also be warned that death might take longer in animals that have been sedated prior to i/v administration of barbiturate.

## CASE 51

**1 What is the most likely species of tapeworm causing this problem?** Rabbits act as an intermediate host for several cestode species, with the definitive hosts being cats, dogs (**51b**) and foxes. Due to the position of the cyst in the soft tissue of the shoulder, the most likely cause is *Coenurus serialis*, the larval stage of the tapeworm *Taenia serialis*. The larvae migrate to the subcutaneous tissues where they form cysts under the skin. These may be palpated as soft, fluctuant swellings.
**2 What is the tapeworm lifecycle?** Infected definitive hosts can defecate tapeworm

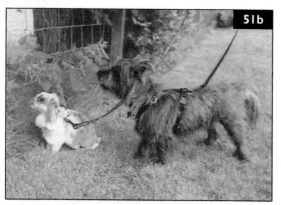

segments containing eggs in their faeces. If defecation occurs on grass used by the rabbit for grazing, then eggs can be ingested by the rabbit. Once ingested, tapeworm eggs hatch in the rabbit's intestines. From there they can migrate to subcutaneous and intramuscular tissues throughout the body and form cysts (**51c**).

**3 What treatment plan do you advise?** If cysts are

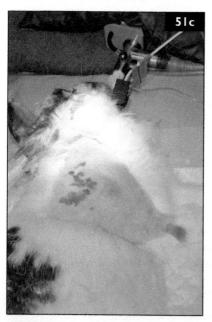

established, surgical removal under a general anaesthetic is required. It is very important that complete removal of the cyst occurs. To try to prevent further cysts from forming, praziquantel can be administered at 5–10 mg/kg p/o, s/c or i/m and repeated in 10 days. It is important to remove cysts prior to treatment being administered otherwise dead tapeworms can cause granulomatous inflammation and foreign body reactions.

**4 How can you prevent rabbits from developing this infection?** To prevent tapeworm infections in rabbits, pastures contaminated with dog, cat or fox faecal material should be avoided. Bedding and hay should be stored hygienically (e.g. in sealed containers) to prevent contamination from infected definitive hosts.

## CASE 52
What essential physical assessments and daily observations of a hospitalized rabbit (52) are required, at least at the beginning of the day, to enable an informed patient assessment? Hospitalized rabbits should receive a physical examination at the beginning of the day at the very least to assess the need for changes in treatment plans. This should include general demeanour and body positioning or mobility of the rabbit, which can be assessed from a distance. Indicators of pain, such as a hunched position or immobility, are particularly important. Essential daily observations should include food intake, urinary output and faecal output (number, size and consistency of droppings). The rabbit should then be placed on an examination table and the following assessments performed; respiratory rate and character, heart rate and rhythm, auscultation and assessment of gut sounds, abdominal palpation, rectal temperature, body weight and hydration status. Other physical assessments will depend on the reason for hospitalization and might include examination of a surgical wound, for example.

## CASE 53
Comment on the use of nitrous oxide in rabbit anaesthesia. Nitrous oxide causes minimal cardiovascular and respiratory depression. It is used to reduce the required concentration of other volatile agents and so reduce the overall degree of blood pressure depression or respiration at a particular depth of anaesthesia. However, nitrous oxide has a relatively low potency in rabbits (high minimum alveolar concentration of anaesthetic). Sixty per cent nitrous oxide will only reduce the concentration of volatile anaesthetic required for maintenance by 0.25–0.5%. Therefore, there is little advantage for its use and, in light of the fact that many rabbits have underlying respiratory disease, it is preferable to use 100% oxygen. Nitrous oxide is not removed by activated charcoal gas scavenging systems, so there are also human health and safety implications.

If used for prolonged periods, 100% oxygen should be administered following cessation of nitrous oxide in order to prevent diffusion hypoxia, where lowered alveolar oxygen tension occurs due to rapid diffusion of nitrous oxide from the blood to the alveoli.

## CASE 54
1 What is the condition shown, and what is the most likely aetiology in this case? Incisor malocclusion. Given the age of the animal, the most likely aetiology is that of a congenital conformational problem, resulting in an excessive length of the mandible relative to the maxilla. This is often referred to as mandibular prognathism, although the actual defect lies in the shortening of the maxilla and is

129

therefore perhaps more correctly described as maxillary brachygnathism (all these terms being borrowed from human dentistry). Unopposed growth and eruption of the mandibular incisors leads to obvious forward protrusion, while the lack of labial occlusal pressure results in a permanent straightening of the tooth. However, the greater curvature of the maxillary incisors, maintained by contact of the labial surfaces with the mandible, causes them to curl caudally into the oral cavity and eventually into the hard palate. The condition has been shown to be an inherited, autosomal, recessive trait, especially in Dwarf and Lop breeds, in particular the Netherland Dwarf. However, all breeds can be affected. Given the hereditary nature of the condition, the rabbit should be neutered or not bred from and any siblings or progeny should be examined.

Alternative aetiologies include dental trauma, inappropriate trimming and acquired malocclusion, the latter being unlikely given the age.

**2 What treatment/management options are available?** Management of the condition involves trimming the teeth using a high-speed burr. In cases of congenital malocclusion (and long-standing acquired cases with straightening of the mandibular incisors), this must be done repeatedly, perhaps as often as every 4–6 weeks, as the teeth can never be brought back into occlusion. However, with care this procedure can be achieved without anaesthesia. The use of nail clippers is contraindicated as this will result in longitudinal fractures, pulp exposure and concussive trauma to the apical germinal tissues.

A permanent solution is extraction. Each surgically loosened tooth is finally pushed into the alveolus before extraction in order to destroy the germinal tissues at the apex. Failure to do so completely may result in the continued growth of an abnormal tooth, as it will fracture below the gingival margin at the time of surgery. The owner should be warned of this possibility at the outset. Radiography should be performed preoperatively to assess the extent of dental disease.

## CASE 55

A 2-year-old rabbit presents with acute onset posterior paresis (55). What are the differential diagnoses? Differential diagnoses include vertebral fracture or luxation secondary to trauma, intervertebral disc disease, spondylosis, meningitis, spinal abscess, encephalitozoonosis, *Baylisascaris procyonis* infestation (cerebrospinal nematodiasis) in the USA, toxoplasmosis, cerebrovascular incident, ingestion of toxins (e.g. heavy metals, pesticides, rodenticides and plant toxins), spinal neoplasia, splay leg and congenital anomalies such as hemivertebrae and kyphosis. The latter two conditions are less likely, as they would present at an earlier age. The rabbit should also be examined for clinical signs associated with systemic disease, as this may cause generalized weakness, which may initially present in the hindlimbs. Systemic disease such as septicaemia, liver failure, renal failure, hepatic lipidosis and cardiovascular disease could potentially have this clinical presentation. Hypokalaemia has been implicated in cases of muscular weakness in rabbits. Myasthenia gravis has been anecdotally reported in the rabbit, with a rapid response noted to i/v edrophonium administration.

## CASE 56

**1 What does the radiograph reveal?** The radiograph shows patchy homogeneous increased lung opacity, with air bronchograms in the caudodorsal lung field. This is an alveolar pattern.

**2 What are your differential diagnoses?** Bronchopneumonia is the most likely diagnosis in a young rabbit. *Pasteurella multocida* should always be considered in respiratory disease in rabbits. This is a commensal organism of the mucous membranes that exhibits pathogenicity when the host's immune defences are compromised. Other bacteria that are often diagnosed in pet rabbits include *Pseudomonas aeruginosa*, *Staphylococcus aureus*, *Bordetella bronchiseptica*, *Mycobacterium bovis*, *M. tuberculosis*, *Moraxella bovis*, *Francisella tularensis*, *Yersinia pestis*, *Chlamydophila* spp. and cilia-associated respiratory (CAR) bacillus. *B. bronchiseptica* and *S. aureus* are thought to act as co-pathogens, although pure cultures have also been isolated from affected rabbits. Some viruses have also been found associated with bronchopneumonia; severe myxomatosis infection can result in haemorrhagic pneumonia and herpesvirus can also be involved. Pulmonary oedema associated with cardiac disease will present with the same radiographic changes but is more likely to occur in older rabbits.

## CASE 57

**Describe how you would auscultate the thorax of a rabbit.** The rabbit should be adequately restrained on the examination table by an assistant, who holds it around the shoulders. The hindquarters are tucked in towards the assistant's abdomen and the rabbit faces away from them. Alternatively, the clinician can restrain the rabbit in this position. The table should have a non-slip surface. The use of a paediatric stethoscope is recommended for thoracic auscultation in rabbits (57). Differentiation between upper and lower respiratory tract sound

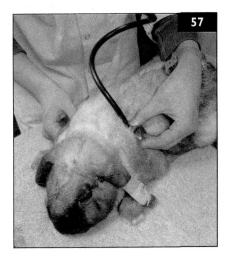

is difficult in this species. The area of auscultation of the lung fields is small in the rabbit and the heart is situated more cranially than in cats and dogs. This should be borne in mind when placing the head of the stethoscope over the thorax. The trachea and sinuses may also be auscultated to determine if sounds originate from the upper respiratory tract. In severe cases, such as an animal with bronchopneumonia, areas with patchy loss of sound and pulmonary rales may be detected. In larger rabbits the thorax may be percussed to detect areas of reduced resonance associated with fluid accumulation or space-occupying lesions such as abscesses or neoplasia.

## CASE 58

**1 Characterize the anaemia from the red cell morphology.** Polychromatic, anisocytotic anaemia.

**2 What stain may be used to differentiate reticulocytes more accurately?** New methylene blue.

**3 What is the most likely cause of this anaemia, and give a differential diagnosis.** Plumbism (lead toxicosis). In this case it occurred because the rabbit gnawed at painted skirting boards in the house. Although currently manufactured house paints do not contain lead salt pigments, in many cases old paint layers are not removed but simply painted over with new paint. The serum lead level in this case was 12.0 µmol/l. Other less frequent differentials for a regenerative anaemia include blood loss due to trauma, intestinal or internal haemorrhage, intravascular haemolysis or severe flea infestation. Chronic disease and neoplasia such as uterine adenocarcinoma are more likely to manifest as a non-regenerative anaemia.

**4 What other haematological and biochemistry abnormalities may occur with this condition?** Lead toxicosis may also manifest in cytoplasmic basophilic stippling, and the regenerative response may lead to the presence of nucleated erythrocytes and metarubricytes on blood smears. Resultant hepatic damage may result in elevations in alkaline phosphatase (ALP), ALT and bilirubin levels.

## CASE 59

**1 What technique is being used in this rabbit (59)?** The rabbit has a nasal catheter in place.

**2 How is it performed, and what are its applications?** A small urinary catheter, 1.0–1.5 mm endotracheal tube or proprietary soft nasogastric tube is premeasured from the nares to the caudal skull and inserted ventrally and medially into the ventral nasal meatus. Application of local anaesthetic drops or gel prior to insertion is advisable. The tube is secured in place on the head using tape or tissue glue. Occasionally, passage of the tube is obstructed by elongated maxillary incisor roots. Bleeding from the turbinates may also occur. This technique can be used to provide supplemental oxygen to rabbits anaesthetized with injectable agents where administering oxygen by mask would be impractical (e.g. for dental surgery). Direct intubation is always preferable, however, and dentistry can generally be carried out with an endotracheal tube in place. Alternatively, volatile anaesthetic agents can be administered by this route. It should be noted, however, that it is not possible to scavenge volatile agents using this route of administration, so there is a risk of operator exposure. A high flow rate of oxygen must be used to create positive pressure within the nasal passages and nasopharynx. The tube can be advanced further to enter the trachea, and this route of endotracheal intubation may be useful in very small rabbits where intubation via the larynx is difficult. There is the potential for introduction of pathogens such as *Pasteurella multocida* from the nasal passages into the lower respiratory tract, and high oxygen flow rates must be used to overcome the resistance to flow with very small tubes.

## CASE 60

**1 What are the major contributing factors to this condition?** The most common contributing factor is a compromised immune system. Stress due to malnutrition, chronic disease, husbandry problems (high ammonia levels), social changes and environmental problems (overheating, poor ventilation) will reduce the host's immune system. Immunosuppression due to corticosteroid therapy or immune system disease will also predispose the rabbit to commensal or opportunistic pathogens. Co-infection with infectious agents that damage the mucocillary escalator (*B. bronchiseptica* and CAR bacillus) will contribute to the severity of the respiratory disease.

**2 How would you treat this rabbit?** Antibacterial treatment of bronchopneumonia should ideally be based on the results of bacterial culture and sensitivity, as resistant bacteria may occur. While waiting for results of bacterial culture, treatment should be started with antibiotics to which *Pasteurella multocida* has been shown to be sensitive and to which *P. multocida* currently has the least resistance. These include penicillin G, chloramphenicol, erythromycin, tetracyclines, fluoroquinolones, novobiocin and nitrofurans. Antibiotics to which *P. multocida* is known to have resistance include lincomycin, clindamycin and, to some degree, streptomycin and sulphonamides. (NB: Many penicillins, erythromycin, lincomycin, clindamycin and streptomycin may be toxic to rabbits, causing GI disturbances, and so these should not be given by the oral route.) In severe infections the use of parenteral, nebulized and topical antibiotics may be indicated. NSAIDs, mucolytics (bromhexine, N-acetyl-cysteine) and humidification are useful in the management of these cases. Assisted feeding and fluid therapy are indicated if anorexia occurs. Any contributing factors should also be addressed.

## CASE 61

Buserelin is licensed for use in rabbits in the UK. What is it indicated for and what is its mode of action? To induce ovulation and improve conception rate in commercial does. It is a synthetic hormone, similar to luteinizing hormone (LH) and follicle-stimulating hormone (FSH), which are produced in the hypothalamus. It stimulates pituitary release of LH and FSH.

## CASE 62

What is the maximum volume per kg body weight that should be administered by s/c injection in rabbits (62)? The maximum volume given by s/c injection depends on the size of the animal and the product to be injected. Irritant products should be avoided where possible. Up to 30 ml/kg body weight of isotonic fluid can be given on either side of the animal as fluid therapy in rabbits.

## CASE 63

1 Describe how you determine the sex of a rabbit. The anogenital distance is slightly greater in males, which have a round preputial opening. Gentle pressure applied above the preputial opening should protrude the penis (63a). Scrotal sacs will be present in mature bucks lateral to the prepuce. Females have an elliptical or slit-like vulval opening (63b). Within a breed, does tend to be slightly larger than bucks, but bucks have broader heads. It is important to recheck the genitalia when a rabbit is anaesthetized for neutering, as incorrect sexing is common.

2 When is the best age to sex rabbit kits? At birth or at weaning (5–8 weeks). In between these ages it is difficult to exteriorize the genitalia by stretching the perineum.

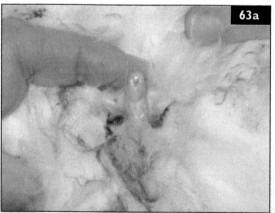

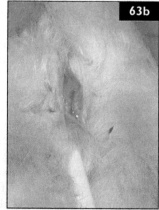

3 At what age do rabbits become sexually mature? 3.5–5 months in the female and 5–8 months in the male. Smaller breeds mature earlier than larger ones. Kits should be separated into single sex groups by 10–12 weeks of age to ensure there is no danger of sibling matings.

## CASE 64

A 2-year-old pet rabbit with diarrhoea is to be hospitalized for fluid therapy. What are the basic housing requirements for hospitalized rabbits? The rabbit should be housed in a cage that is easy to disinfect and has non-slip flooring. This can easily be achieved using standard dog or cat stainless steel cages with newspaper as flooring (64). Ideally, the animal should

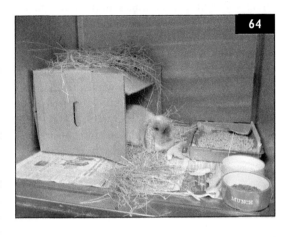

be kept in a quiet area or, if available, a separate ward, away from the noise of barking dogs and cats, because rabbits are prey species and are quickly stressed. A hide area is easily provided using a cardboard box at the back of the cage. If the rabbit is litter trained, a litter tray with wood or paper-based litter should be provided. It is important to feed the rabbit its usual diet and the owner should be asked to provide this information prior to hospitalization. Fresh meadow hay and access to water in a recognizable form to the rabbit should be available at all times. A supply of good quality feed should also be available. Rapid changes to the diet must be avoided, as this may induce further GI upset and result in anorexia. Ill rabbits often favour fresh greens over a dry diet and a small quantity of fresh vegetables and grass should be made available.

## CASE 65

1 In relation to rabbit digestive physiology, what do the terms digestible fibre and indigestible fibre refer to? Fibre is provided by the components of the plant cell walls that are ingested, and it includes cellulose, hemicelluloses, pectins and lignin. Fibre can be divided into digestible/fermentable (soluble) and indigestible (insoluble) components, based on particle size. The digestible fibre refers to the proportion of this material that is directed into the caecum and acts as a substrate for fermentation by the resident microorganisms. In general the digestible fibre is

composed of particles that are less than 0.3 mm in size. Indigestible fibre consists of larger particles (>0.35 mm) of plant cell wall material that pass through the GI system without entering the caecum. This type of fibre is mostly made up of lignin and cellulose.

**2 Discuss the health benefits of a diet high in indigestible fibre.** A diet high in indigestible fibre encourages natural foraging behaviour and thereby prevents boredom and associated behavioural conditions. It also provides optimal (mainly lateral) mandibular chewing movements and dental wear, stimulates and maintains gut motility, stimulates appetite, and encourages the practice of caecotrophy.

**3 Other than hay, what foods provide a source of fibre?** Fresh grass is an excellent source of fibre, as are garden weeds, tree leaves and bark. If such natural sources are unavailable or provided only in limited amounts, a variety of fresh vegetables can provide an additional source of fibre. Most concentrate foods do provide a fibre source; however, the manufacturing process of these feeds can alter the digestibility of the fibre provided.

## CASE 66

A 2-year-old rabbit presents with a recent history of progressive loss of vision associated with bilateral cataracts (66). What are the causes of cataract formation in the rabbit, and what advice would you give the owner on the possibility of restoring sight? Congenital cataracts in young rabbits and cataract formation following lens rupture due to infection with *Encephalitozoon cuniculi*. Diabetes mellitus is a rare condition in rabbits and is not associated with cataract formation. In the absence of any other eye disease, bilateral cataract is likely to be primary and may be suitable for surgical lens removal by phacoemulsification and aspiration. Other eye conditions should be excluded before performing such surgery. This should include serological screening for *E. cuniculi* infection and ocular ultrasonography to exclude any posterior segment disease. If surgery is not an option, then the rabbit should be able to live a satisfactory lifestyle in a controlled environment without sight, provided the home layout remains constant and there is no competition from companion rabbits.

## CASE 67

**1 What is the significance of the elevated value, and what is the likely cause?**
Reference ranges for blood calcium values for rabbits vary widely between different laboratories and published sources. These are normally based on the distribution of normal values seen by that laboratory. However, high blood calcium levels, even as high as 4.6 mmol/l (18.4 mg/dl), are generally regarded as normal in the rabbit. Absorption of dietary calcium is extremely effective in rabbits, with the excess

being excreted via the kidneys. High dietary calcium intake is the likely cause of the levels seen in this rabbit. Rabbit pellets based on lucerne (alfalfa) will have a high calcium content, as will a variety of greens, including dandelions, broccoli, kale, watercress and parsley. While not a problem in itself, high calcium intake will lead to high levels being excreted in the urine. In some rabbits, poor water intake, inactivity and obesity or other disease predisposes to the formation of bladder sludge (crystalluria) due to the sedimentation of calcium carbonate and oxalate crystals, which may be a cause of discomfort and dysuria.

## CASE 68

**1 Describe the oestrous cycle of the rabbit.** Rabbits are reflex ovulators with no regular oestrous cycle, although receptiveness of the doe towards a buck does follow a cyclic rhythm. Follicles develop in response to increased follicular stimulating hormone (FSH) and produce increased oestrogen levels. Waves of follicles develop and regress on the ovaries, and this is reflected by periods of receptivity, usually for 12–14 days, followed by 2–4 days of non-receptivity. This can vary, and some does become receptive every 4–6 days during the breeding season (January to October in the northern hemisphere). Other factors such as photoperiod, nutritional status, environmental temperature and presence of a male will also influence this cyclic rhythm. Ovulation occurs approximately 10 hours after mating.

**2 How should a buck and doe be introduced for mating?** Does are highly territorial, so the doe should always be taken to the buck for mating. An alternative is to introduce the doe and buck on neutral territory. If the doe does not accept the buck's advances within a few minutes and becomes aggressive, they should be separated, then reintroduced at 12–24 hour intervals until mating occurs.

**3 What is the gestation period and what methods of pregnancy diagnosis are possible in the rabbit?** 30–32 days. Fetal palpation is possible from 14 days. Ultrasonography (from day 8 onwards) and radiography (from day 11 onwards) may also be used and are both reliable. It should be noted that fetal resorption can occur up to 20 days post mating.

## CASE 69

**1 Identify the tools and describe their uses.** The rodent mouth gag and cheek dilators in **69a** are shown in use (**69c**). They are essential to maximize access to the oral cavity in the anaesthetized patient, allowing full examination and reducing the risk of trauma when using power tools.

Molar cutters (far left) are used to clip spurs from the cheek teeth. However, they are not suitable for reducing exposed crown length (transverse sectioning of the entire tooth), which may result in fracture or trauma to the apical or periodontal

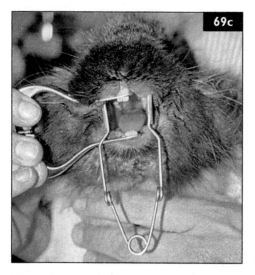

69c

tissues, already compromised by ongoing dental disease. The ends of the Crossley molar elevators/ luxators (second from left) are orientated perpendicular to the shaft of the instrument to enable insertion into the periodontal space of a cheek tooth. One end is flattened longitudinally for the lingual and buccal aspects, and the other transversely for the rostral and caudal aspects. The periodontal ligament is ablated and the loosened tooth then grasped with the molar extraction forceps (third from left), the ends of which are again turned at right angles to the shaft. The tooth can then be manipulated in such a way as to crush the germinal tissues (to prevent regrowth) and then be removed.

The shape of each 'blade' of the Crossley incisor elevators/luxators (second from right) is designed to match the lateral profile of the primary incisors. One end has greater curvature than the other, comparable to that of the upper and lower incisors, respectively. The instrument is used to ablate the medial and lateral periodontal ligaments of these teeth prior to extraction.

**2 Which of the tools in 69b would you choose for inclusion in your dental kit? Explain your preference.** Molar rasps (69b) are intended for gently smoothing the occlusal surfaces and edges of the molariform arcades. They should not be used to reduce exposed crown length. Two types are shown. The one on the left has deep transverse grooves that 'lock' into the transverse enamel ridges of the cheek teeth, which can then be subjected to excessive distractive forces that will tear the periodontal ligament. The sharp diamond coating on the other instrument is more finely abrasive and therefore more suitable for its limited purpose.

## CASE 70

**1 What underlying condition would you suspect?** Cutaneous asthenia due to a collagen defect similar to Ehlers-Danlos syndrome, a group of inherited connective tissue defects characterized in animals by skin fragility, skin hypermobility and poor wound healing.

**2 How would you confirm your diagnosis?** Skin biopsy and electron microscopy to examine dermal collagen fibrils. Histological examination may be unrewarding.

3 **How would you treat this rabbit?** There is no specific treatment. Suturing of the skin often leads to further tearing and damage. Cyanoacrylate tissue glue may be more successful at closing wounds. The rabbit should be housed and managed in such a way as to avoid skin trauma (e.g. avoid handling unless absolutely necessary). If lesions become severe, euthanasia should be considered.

## CASE 71

**What volume of blood can be safely collected at any one time in a 2 kg pet rabbit, and how is this calculated?** The maximum volume removed at any one time should not exceed 10% of the circulating blood volume. Total blood volume in a healthy rabbit ranges between 5.5% and 7% of body weight. Therefore, in a 2 kg rabbit the total blood volume ranges between 110 ml and 140 ml and the maximum volume of blood that may be safely taken is 11–14 ml. A slightly lower volume may be prudent for juveniles, elderly or debilitated animals or suspected anaemic cases.

## CASE 72

1 **What are your differential diagnoses for bilateral nasal discharge in a rabbit?** Differential diagnoses can be divided into infectious and non-infectious causes.

*Infectious causes* could include:
- Bacterial – *Pasteurella multocida, Bordetella bronchiseptica, Pseudomonas, Staphylococcus, Treponema cuniculi*
- Viral – myxoma virus, herpes virus (rare)
- Fungal – granuloma formation, e.g. *Aspergillus* spp.

*Non-infectious causes* could include:
- Bilateral dental disease from the maxillary incisors and/or 1st premolar roots disrupting the nasal lacrimal duct, dental abscesses, elongation and infection of maxillary cheek teeth roots leading to secondary infection of the nasal cavity.
- Dacryocystitis infection draining into the nasal passage.
- Trauma – blunt force, predators, secondary to endotracheal intubation.
- Neoplasia – carcinoma and adenocarcinoma have been reported resulting in destruction of the nasal turbinates, but these often present initially with unilateral discharge.
- Foreign body – hay, hair or grass seeds have been reported, although these usually affect only one side of the nasal passage.
- Respiratory irritants – smoke, dust and high ammonia levels can make the nasal mucosa more susceptible to secondary infections.
- Allergy – rare.

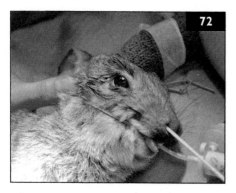

**2 What diagnostic tests could you perform?** Diagnostic tests include blood sampling for routine haematology and serum biochemistry, deep nasal swabs (72); for bacterial and fungal culture and sensitivity, cytology; nasolacrimal flush, radiographic examination, rhinoscopic examination with nasal mucosal biopsies and CT scan.

## CASE 73

**1 What could this increase in radiopacity represent?** The tympanic bullae are normally air-filled structures. An increase in the radiopacity as in the radiograph may indicate the presence of fluid or soft tissues such as cellular debris, exudates and neoplastic tissue.

**2 What diagnostic modality would provide further detail to assess the bullae?** Computed tomography (CT) is a useful modality for examination of the bony structures of the skull and for assessment of the tympanic bullae, tympanic membranes and external ear canal.

**3 What is the most likely diagnosis?** Given the rabbit's history and clinical signs, the most likely diagnosis is unilateral otitis media with associated otitis interna. This problem may occur secondary to chronic otitis externa or, as suspected in this case, as a result of upper respiratory pathogens entering the affected bulla via the Eustachian tube.

**4 In the event that medical treatment is ineffective, are there any surgical options for treatment of such a case?** Bulla osteotomy is indicated in cases of severe refractory otitis media. The success of this procedure is variable, but some surgeons have reported good success rates with this technique. Both ventral and lateral approaches to the bulla have been described in rabbits. The bulla is accessed and samples of the contents should be collected for culture and cytology. Following curettage, the soft tissues over the bulla are closed routinely.

**5 What postoperative complications could be expected with this technique?** Postoperative complications associated with bulla osteotomy include cellulitis, abscess formation, vestibular dysfunction, facial muscle contracture, facial nerve palsy, Horner's syndrome and, rarely, transient hypoglossal nerve palsy. As with other surgical procedures, the patient's gastrointestinal function needs to be supported in the postoperative period to prevent ileus and appropriate analgesia provided.

## CASE 74
**What advice would you give to this owner on how to deal with this problem?**
Rabbits thump their feet to alert other members of the group that there is danger
and that they should retreat to the burrow. It is highly likely that this rabbit was
scared, either on one evening or a succession of evenings by an external stimulus
(e.g. the presence of a predator within the garden or near the hutch, fireworks or a
thunderstorm, or a fear-eliciting odour). The ongoing nature of this problem may
not mean that the threat is present every evening. An intermittent exposure or even
a one-off experience can lead the animal to anticipate the threat when it finds itself
in the same situation again (i.e. in the hutch in the early hours of the morning).

A resolution to the problem is more likely if the owner can pinpoint the stressor,
but she should consider moving the rabbit to a more secure location at night. A garage
or utility room provides the obvious answer. Failing that, the owner should consider
covering up the hutch with tarpaulin at night to enable the rabbit to feel more secure.

## CASE 75
**1 What is the likely cause of the urine colour?** Urine pigments (urochromes)
colour rabbit urine, resulting in normal urine being a variety of colours. Pigments
occur in the urine as a result of excretion of ingested plant pigment, breakdown
of endogenous compounds (such as porphyrins, flavins and bile pigments) and
by ingested foods affecting the metabolism of bile pigments (e.g. cauliflower and
cabbage). All these colour variations are normal, but they can mimic haematuria.
A normal urine sample may be differentiated from haematuria by a simple urine
dipstick test or microscopy of urine sediment. A small amount of albumin is normal
in rabbit urine.
**2 What is the likely cause of the turbidity?** Normal rabbit urine can be turbid
and a fine sediment is often evident if it is left to settle. Fine calcium carbonate,
ammonium magnesium phosphate and calcium oxalate crystals are found in
normal rabbit urine due to their unique calcium metabolism. Excess calcium is
excreted in the urine and crystals are especially evident in rabbits fed calcium-rich
foods such as Lucerne/alfalfa hay or pellets.

## CASE 76
*Pasteurella multocida* is commonly involved in respiratory disease in rabbits. How
can this infection be controlled and prevented? Serological screening for *P. multocida*
and barrier housing have been used to establish *Pasteurella*-free colonies in laboratory
rabbits and large breeding facilities. However, pet rabbits are unlikely to originate
from *Pasteurella*-free sources and a high percentage of normal healthy rabbits carry
this bacterium as a commensal organism in their respiratory tract. Prevalence increases

with age and clinical signs depend on the immune status of the host, virulence, and strain of bacterium involved. Therefore, carrying out serological screening for *P. multocida*, quarantining positive animals and treating infected rabbits is likely to have little effect on the control of *Pasteurella* in a multi-rabbit household. Careful attention to any contributing factors will decrease the individual's susceptibility to infection. Common contributing factors include stress due to malnutrition, chronic disease, husbandry problems (high ammonia levels), social changes and environmental problems (overheating, poor ventilation). Immunosuppression due to corticosteroid therapy or immune system disease will also predispose the rabbit to this infection. Excellent husbandry practices, such as good ventilation and hygiene, and reducing any stressors will reduce the incidence of this disease. New animals should be quarantined and observed for respiratory signs prior to being introduced to other pet rabbits. Vaccines have been developed against *P. multocida* in laboratory rabbits, although none are currently available for prevention of pasteurellosis in pet rabbits in the UK.

## CASE 77

**1 What would your approach be to this case?** A full clinical examination (including assessment of teeth) will often identify an obvious source of pain preventing activity and grooming. Osteoarthritis and spondylosis are common problems in the older rabbit and may be confirmed by radiography. Sedation or general anaesthesia is generally required for diagnostic spinal radiographs, and pre-anaesthetic bloods would be recommended in an older inactive patient such as this due to the risk of underlying renal or other systemic disease.

**2 What supportive treatment would you recommend?** Rabbits rarely show obvious signs of pain, but analgesia is indicated for any potentially painful condition. NSAIDs such as meloxicam are effective in many cases and generally well tolerated. However, if used long-term, doses should be reduced as clinical signs improve to the lowest effective dose in order to reduce the risk of side effects, especially in the older patient. The addition of alternative analgesics such as tramadol may also be considered for some rabbits although effectiveness seems to vary depending on the individual. Owners should also be encouraged to modify the rabbit's environment to reduce opportunities to jump or climb and to prevent the rabbit slipping on smooth surfaces.

## CASE 78

**What advice would you give to the client?** The sudden development of aggression in rabbits is quite common and is often confusing for owners who make the assumption that neutering their pet ensures that there will never be any aggression problems. A veterinary examination is advisable in the first instance to ensure that the rabbit is not in any discomfort or obvious underlying pain.

Neutering does not prevent aggression developing in any animal; it affects only behaviours that are under hormonal control. These include primary sexual behaviours, such as mounting, and aggressive disputes towards a rabbit of the same sex over a rabbit of the opposite sex. Neutering does not calm an animal down, affect its personality or make it more docile. It has been suggested that neutering a nervous animal can make it more likely to show aggression, as sexual hormones that promote confidence are reduced.

To a certain extent, territorial behaviour is motivated by hormones and can be seen to increase at certain times of the year (e.g. during the main rabbit breeding season from January to August). Aggression towards the owner in a neutered rabbit can develop suddenly and may be linked to a change in environment, a change in routine or the rabbit feeling under threat. It is worth ensuring that the owner has washed their hands before they handle the rabbit; even rubbing them in some of the rabbit's dirty litter may help.

If the problem still continues, it is worth considering the rabbit's environment to see if the rabbit could be feeling threatened by the manner in which the owner approaches. Sometimes, rabbits have had a fright from something that owners unwittingly do and then lose all confidence in their interactions. The owner should be encouraged to combine the hand feeding of some of the rabbit's favourite treats with some handling.

There is often misinterpretation of behavioural patterns by owners. If a rabbit is reported to be building a nest, this could be due to plucking the fur from the chest and using it to line a corner of the hutch or cage, or due to plucking fur from herself in a manner that might suggest over-grooming. It is possible that the rabbit is not plucking fur from herself, but has moved her bedding around to create a shallow indent that looks like a nest.

It would be quite unusual for a neutered doe to build a nest, akin to the nest built by a nursing doe, but there are does that may feel threatened and, as they are unable to dig a burrow, consequently move all their bedding to create a shallow indent and lie in that. Rabbits can indulge in over-grooming if they are living in a stressful environment or if there is a lack of environmental stimulation.

## CASE 79
**Identify these rabbit breeds**

a Angora
b New Zealand White
c English Lop

d Netherland Dwarf
e English
f Dutch

## CASE 80

**What are the common venepuncture sites in the rabbit, and what are their relative advantages/disadvantages?** There are several different sites that may be used for venepuncture in the rabbit. The lateral saphenous vein can be found located across the lateral aspect of the tibia. The vein is relatively mobile and an assistant is required to hold the rabbit in lateral recumbency and raise the vein just below the stifle joint. This site should not be used in fractious or easily stressed animals without prior sedation. Alternatively, the rabbit may be restrained in sternal recumbency and the hindlimb extended down over the edge of the table to give easy access to this venepuncture site. Large haematomas can occur at this site if adequate pressure is not applied following sampling.

The marginal ear vein is easily accessible, even in the smaller breeds, although only relatively small volumes of blood can be collected. Blood sample collection from this site is more difficult in debilitated animals. Damage to the vein may result

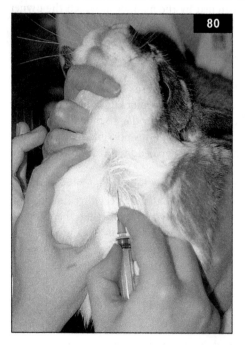

in thrombosis and skin sloughing over the affected area. This potential complication is commonest in the smaller rabbit breeds. Haematoma formation and subcutaneous bruising is easily visible at this site and may displease the owner.

Rabbits have large paired jugular veins, which are easily located, except in extremely obese animals or rabbits with large dewlaps. This site readily yields a large volume of blood and may be used without sedation in calm rabbits, following application of a topical local anaesthetic cream (80).

The cephalic vein is easily accessible in most rabbits, the exception being those with short forelimbs, where it may prove difficult to identify this vein. Collection of blood without sedation is relatively easy at this site.

## CASE 81

**1 What is the most likely diagnosis in this case, and what are the possible aetiologies?** The condition shown is hypopyon. The marked corneal vascularization is suggestive of a chronic condition of at least a week's duration. Possible aetiologies include uveitis secondary to penetrating trauma, systemic infection or immune-mediated disease and lymphoma. The latter cannot be excluded definitively without cytological examination. In the absence of a history of foreign body penetration, a lens-induced uveitis associated with *Encephalitozoon cuniculi* infection and lens capsule rupture is most likely in this case.

**2 How would you investigate and treat this condition?** Further investigation might include serological screening for *E. cuniculi* infection, ultrasonography to rule out involvement of the posterior structures of the eye and visual response testing to demonstrate the presence or absence of visual function. Treatment in this case consists of surgical lens removal. If the prognosis for the restoration of sight is hopeless, enucleation would be the preferred option. Enucleation in the rabbit carries the risk of damage to the orbital sinus and significant haemorrhage.

## CASE 82

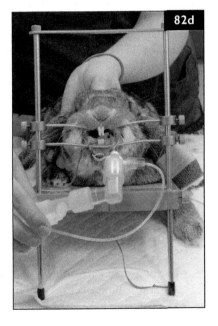

**1 Describe the dentistry applications for the instruments shown (82a, b, c).** The hand-piece (arrowed) of the foot-operated power equipment (82c) rotates the burr (82a) or diamond disc (82b) at high speed. The burrs can be used to trim incisors that have overgrown as a result of congenital or acquired malocclusion and also to grind down elongated cheek teeth in cases of acquired dental disease. Because of its size and orientation, the disc is only suitable for reduction of incisor length.

**2 What precautions are required for their safe use in each case?** The major concern is avoidance of damage to the surrounding soft tissue. Many burrs and discs are supplied with guards that enclose all but the section of the circumference required to contact the tooth. Wooden or metal tongue depressors are also invaluable to shield and retract tissues. For cheek teeth, a general anaesthetic and use of a gag (hand held or table-top) and cheek dilators is essential (82d). Many docile rabbits will tolerate incisor trimming with only

145

moderate physical restraint (e.g. wrapping in a towel and careful retraction of the lips). However, many clinicians prefer sedation, especially when using the diamond disc as there is a significant risk of injury to the rabbit should it move during the procedure. Another important consideration is dissipation of the considerable heat that is generated when grinding teeth. High-speed drills require a continuous water spray, whereas frequent application of water from a soaked cotton bud is sufficient for low-speed burrs. Failure to do so can result in pulpitis and pulp necrosis.

## CASE 83

**1 What advice would you give a client keen to keep pet rabbits as to the ideal number and sex combination (83)?** Rabbits are highly social animals; ideally they should always be kept with a companion. The most stable combination and best pair-bond is a neutered buck and a neutered doe, preferably purchased from the same litter so there is no issue of introduction. Two neutered does or neutered bucks may live together well, but the pairing is generally less stable and fighting may occur. Intact bucks invariably fight, often causing severe injuries, as can intact does. Same-sex pairs are most successful if they are litter mates. Where it is only possible to keep a single rabbit, the owner must be prepared to devote significant time to interacting with the rabbit and providing companionship.

**2 How should unfamiliar rabbits be introduced to each other?** New rabbits should be introduced on neutral territory and monitored closely at all times. Hide boxes should be provided, preferably with one more than the number of rabbits present. For the first few days to weeks, rabbits should be physically separated within sight and scent of each other when unsupervised, as serious fighting may occur. Once the rabbits are ready to be fully introduced, any existing territory should be thoroughly cleaned and deodorized as completely as possible, and the rabbits returned there and again monitored closely.

**3 Should rabbits be kept with guinea pigs?** It is not recommended to keep guinea pigs and rabbits together for the following reasons:

- Rabbits can often bully guinea pigs and injure them by kicking or biting. If housed together, the guinea pig should have an escape area that only it can access to avoid this.
- Both bucks and does may mount the guinea pig, causing it stress and possible injury.
- Rabbits can carry *Bordetella bronchiseptica* in their nasal passages, which is non-pathogenic to the rabbit but potentially pathogenic to the guinea pig.
- Guinea pigs have an absolute requirement for high levels of vitamin C and, if fed a rabbit pelleted diet, sufficient levels will not be provided.

However, there are always exceptions to any rule and there are some rabbits and guinea pigs that appear to form a strong pair-bond. If kept together, size disparity should be kept to a minimum if possible.

## CASE 84

**Why is castration recommended in male rabbits (84), and what is the recommended age for this procedure?** Castration is recommended in male rabbits for the following reasons:

- to prevent unwanted pregnancies
- to reduce aggression, particularly between companion males
- to reduce hypersexual behaviour
- to reduce territorial urine marking
- in older bucks, because of trauma (commonly males will attack each other's genitals), neoplasia or infection (orchitis or epididymitis)
- in order to allow housing with a female (preferably spayed) or other males (also castrated).

The procedure is generally recommended any time after 4 months of age, when male rabbits can become fertile, but ideally around 5 months old.

## CASE 85

**Describe how you would collect blood from the marginal ear vein of a pet rabbit.** The marginal ear vein is situated on the dorso-lateral edge of the rabbit's pinna and is easily accessible. Care should be taken not to confuse this vessel with the large central artery, which, if punctured, may result in thrombosis and subsequent sloughing of the skin. The hair over the vein should be

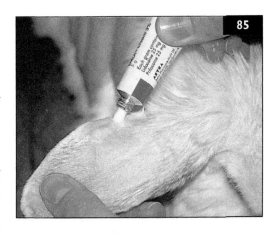

carefully clipped to aid visualization. Exercise caution with clipping the fur, as rabbit skin is thin and easily torn. A topical local anaesthetic cream should be applied 15–20 minutes prior to venepuncture to desensitize the area and reduce the risk of the rabbit making a sudden movement as the needle enters the vein (85).

An assistant should restrain the rabbit and raise the vein near the base of the ear. Rub or tap the area to dilate the vein and swab with alcohol. Use a 25–27 gauge needle with a 1 ml syringe. This may be heparinized depending on the sample required. Insert the needle into the vein and apply gentle negative pressure on the syringe to obtain a sample. Once finished, apply digital pressure to the puncture site for a few minutes to avoid haematoma formation or haemorrhage.

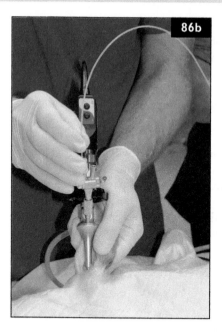

86b

## CASE 86

**1 What is the likely diagnosis?** Bilateral ear base abscesses as a result of otitis externa. The infection pockets in the distal vertical part of the external ear canal, causing the canal and overlying skin to protrude. The infection may be localized to the external ear canal, or can perforate the tympanic membrane causing both an otitis media and externa.

**2 How would you confirm your diagnosis?** Visualization of purulent material in the external ear canal and microscopic examination of cytological samples will confirm the presence of infection. To determine whether the tympanic membrane is intact, CT is the imaging modality of choice, achieving excellent images of the tympanic bullae. Only advanced disease and associated bony changes are likely to be evident with radiographic imaging techniques.

**3 What treatment options could be offered to the owner?** Medical treatment is often advocated in rabbits with otitis media, but it yields poor results and is not therefore recommended. Aural endoscopy under anaesthesia can be used in cases with intact tympanic membranes (as confirmed by CT evaluation) to flush the ear canal to the level of the tympanic membrane and suction any debris (**86b**). Where there is marked dilation of the distal vertical ear canal, with or without an intact tympanum, surgery may be required, as debris and infection is likely to continue to pool here. Surgical options include lateral wall resection where only a partial ear canal ablation (PECA) is performed. Some surgeons prefer a total ear canal ablation (TECA), while a lateral bulla osteotomy may be indicated if infection has ruptured the tympanic membrane and is present in the tympanic bulla.

## CASE 87

**1 What is the lifespan for a pet rabbit?** Rabbits usually live for 8–10 years, but some individuals may live significantly longer.

**2 What common problems are seen in geriatric rabbits?** Osteoarthritis, spondylosis, renal disease, cardiovascular disease and neoplasia are all commonly seen in older rabbits. Any pre-existing problems such as dental disease or cataracts may also progress with age and require careful management.

**3 What preventive healthcare advice would you give for the geriatric rabbit?** Health checks at least twice yearly are recommended to detect any problems at an early stage. Owners should be advised that signs of disease can be subtle and attention should be paid to any changes in behaviour, appetite, thirst, urine and faecal output and activity levels. Regular monitoring of body weight on a weekly basis can also be a useful tool.

# CASE 88

**1 Describe how you would administer fluid therapy to this animal?** Fluid therapy is best administered intravenously or via the intraosseous route. In dehydrated animals, peripheral veins become markedly constricted and i/v catheter placement is more difficult. This is exacerbated in extremely small animals, such as Dwarf breeds, where visualization of peripheral veins is more difficult, even in healthy rabbits. Intravenous catheter placement is achieved using the marginal ear vein, the jugular vein, the lateral saphenous vein or the cephalic vein. Long-term use of the marginal ear vein may cause sloughing, and sedation may be required for the jugular vein. Placement technique is as for other species. An Elizabethan collar can be used for a short period to prevent the rabbit from chewing or removing the catheter, although this may be poorly tolerated in some rabbits and can be stressful to the animal. Use of a topical local anaesthetic cream is recommended prior to catheter placement. If placement of an indwelling catheter is not possible, an intraosseous catheter should be used. This is placed aseptically in the greater trochanter of the femur or the tibial crest. Sedation and local anaesthesia is required and the technique is as in other species. Alternatively, subcutaneous (s/c) or intraperitoneal (i/p) routes may be used; however, subcutaneous absorption of fluids is likely to be slow in a debilitated animal. With intraperitoneal injections there is a risk of iatrogenic organ puncture, particularly of the bladder or caecum.

**2 What type of fluids would you use and at what flow rate?** The decision on what type of fluid therapy to select is based on the same fluid therapy principles as in other mammals. A crystalloid should be used in this case. To calculate fluid flow rates the rabbit should be weighed. Daily maintenance fluid requirements are 75–100 ml/kg/day. Dehydration deficits are added to this as a percentage of body weight, based on clinical signs of dehydration. Shock fluid volumes of 100 ml/kg may be administered over 60 minutes. As a general rule, assume 10% dehydration for debilitated animals. Replace 50% of the fluid deficit in the first 12 hours and the remainder (plus maintenance and concurrent losses) within 48–72 hours. A syringe driver or flow pump should be used to deliver the measured quantity

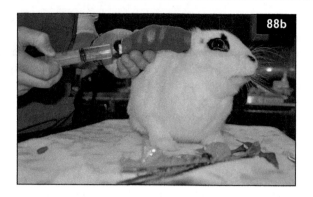

of fluid over a period of time, since fluid volumes may be very small, especially in smaller breeds (88b).

## CASE 89

**List your differential diagnoses for subcutaneous facial swellings in rabbits.** Abscess/cellulitis, due to an external fight wound, associated with dental disease or via bacteraemic spread; myxomatosis; Shope fibroma (USA); neoplasia (lipoma, lymphoma, fibroma and other neoplasms); cuterebriasis (USA); tapeworm larval cysts (*C. serialis*); impacted scent gland; haematoma or seroma; salivary gland cyst; oedema secondary to bite or sting.

## CASE 90

**1 What is your diagnosis?** Atrial fibrillation. The p waves are absent, notably seen on lead I. Lead II shows only small oscillating waves. The QRS complexes have a normal shape but the interval between successive QRS complexes is irregular. The interval between beats two and three and five and six is prolonged in comparison with the other beats on the ECG trace, and this is because of intermittent AV block.
**2 How would you treat this condition?** This is a severe arrhythmia, which occurs with severe heart disease, including congestive heart failure. The congestive heart failure must be controlled. Treatment in this case consisted of furosemide (1 mg/kg i/m q6h). The rabbit died 24 hours later and the owner declined postmortem examination. Digoxin may be used to slow the ventricular rate. This drug has been used in pet rabbits and anecdotal dose rates of 0.005–0.01 mg/kg orally every 12–24 hours have been described. Toxic side effects have been noted in rabbits associated with anorexia and gastrointestinal stasis. Ideally, serum drug levels should be measured following several days of therapy, with samples being taken 6–7 hours post drug dosing.

# CASE 91

**1 What is seen in the radiograph?** A radiodense oval structure which is likely situated in the bladder and likely to be a cystic calculus (**91b**). A lateral abdominal radiographic view should confirm the position of the calculus within the bladder and, as the kidneys are often concurrently affected, these should also be evaluated for calculi. Alternatively an ultrasonographic examination of the entire urinary tract can be performed.

**2 Describe the surgical management of this case.** A cystotomy is indicated for surgical removal of the calculus. Prior to surgery full urinalysis and urine culture should be performed to rule out concurrent infection as well as serum biochemistry and haematology to assess renal function. The technique in rabbits is similar to that in other species. Closure of the bladder is achieved using partial thickness continuous, inverting absorbable monofilament sutures. Closure of the abdomen is routine, using monofilament absorbable suture material.

**3 What postoperative care is indicated?** Analgesia should be provided pre- and postoperatively until the dysuria has resolved and the rabbit is eating satisfactorily. Secondary bacterial cystitis is commonly associated with urolithiasis, so a course of systemic antibiotics may be indicated based on results of urine culture and sensitivity. Diuresis is essential and fluid therapy should be continued postoperatively along with close monitoring of urination. A good quality high-fibre diet should be offered to encourage a return to normal appetite post surgery. Recurrence of urolithiasis is common, so repeat radiography, urine analysis and serum biochemistry and haematology sampling are advisable. General dietary advice to help prevent recurrence should consist of provision of *ad libitum* grass/hay diet, with a reduction in concentrates. However, it should be noted that experimentally, high dietary calcium alone does not induce calculus formation. Hydrating the patient is important in reducing the build-up of large numbers of crystal deposits within the bladder. Weight reduction and increased exercise should also be encouraged.

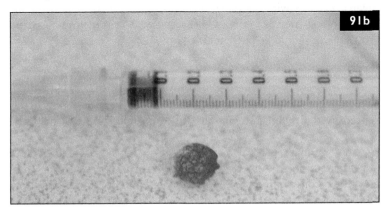

## CASE 92

**1 What further diagnostic tests would you perform?** Routine haematology should be performed to confirm the presence of anaemia, determine whether it is regenerative or non-regenerative and assess the severity. PCV and TP values should be recorded to ascertain whether there has been haemorrhage (reduced PCV and TP) or haemolysis (reduced PCV, normal TP). Severe dehydration may mask anaemia and hypoproteinaemia.

**2 What is your likely diagnosis, and how would you confirm this?** Lead toxicity is more common in house rabbits, where access to lead sources such as lead-based paint or lead pipes is more likely. The classic blood picture includes nucleated red blood cells, hypochromasia, poikilocytosis and cytoplasmic basophilic stippling. Heteropenia, lymphocytosis and a reduced haematocrit may also be seen. Blood lead levels are elevated (>1.45 umol/l). Radiography of the GI tract should be performed to ascertain if there is an enteric lead source. However, the absence of a metallic foreign body does not rule out lead toxicosis; ingested lead may already have been systemically absorbed or not be in an easily visible form (e.g. paint).

**3 What treatment is indicated?** Removal of any GI lead if present radiographically is difficult in the rabbit and treatment usually consists of chelation therapy with sodium calcium edetate (CaEDTA) (27.5 mg/kg s/c q6h) for 5 days on, 5 days off then retest blood lead levels. The CaEDTA should be diluted at a ratio of 1 ml of CaEDTA to 4 ml of sterile water prior to injection. Chelation may be repeated if necessary. CaEDTA acts by forming a stable, water-soluble lead complex that is excreted by the kidneys. As lead can cause renal tubular necrosis, monitoring of renal parameters and maintenance of hydration status are important in preventing further tubular damage and resultant renal failure. Motility modifiers such as metoclopramide, ranitidine or cisapride may also be indicated if ileus is present and to aid excretion of lead from the GI tract. General supportive care should be instigated in cases with anorexia and ileus. If the haematocrit is significantly decreased, a blood transfusion may be necessary. Access to lead-based paint or other lead sources should be prevented.

## CASE 93

**List the measures that can be taken in a veterinary practice to minimize the stress experienced by the rabbit patient.** The following measures can help minimize stress:

- Separate waiting area away from predators, or rabbit consultations scheduled for different times of day to cats, dogs and ferrets.
- Dedicated consultation room, or examination table cleaned and deodorized if previous patient was a predator.

- Handwashing after handling predators before handling the rabbit.
- Change of consulting coat by clinicians if they have previously been handling predators.
- Non-slip examination table.
- Separate hospitalization area away from sight, sound and smell of predators.
- Provision of hide areas in the hospital cage.
- Provision of a familiar diet and water source.
- Minimal handling and manipulation.
- Dim lighting in hospital cage area.
- Minimization of noise (e.g. loud conversations, sudden bangs and crashes).

## CASE 94

**1 How do rabbits thermoregulate?** The main thermoregulatory mechanism in rabbits is via their large ears. These contain a large arteriovenous anastomotic system, allowing effective heat dissipation or conservation via vasodilation or vasoconstriction. Glands in the nasal mucosa that moisten inspired air also have a role in thermoregulation. The dense fur of rabbits is a highly effective insulator. Rabbits are unable to sweat or pant and thus their capacity to lose body heat is limited. Rabbits do not possess brown fat and they shiver when very cold.

**2 How do they cope with extremes of cold and heat?** Rabbits in the wild naturally retreat into their burrows to escape extremes of temperature. They do not cope well with very cold, wet weather if there is no dry shelter. If provided with plenty of bedding and dry shelter, they can easily survive sub-zero temperatures. Extremes of heat are generally more of a problem to rabbits and they succumb rapidly to heat stress. A rise of body temperature to above 40.5 °C can rapidly be fatal.

## CASE 95

**1 What situations can lead to this procedure being necessary, and how can you assess if kits require hand rearing?** Rabbit kits can require hand rearing if they are true orphans due to maternal death, or because of mismothering or lactational failure of the doe. It is important to remember that does only suckle their kittens 1–2 times every 24 hours, at night, for a period of only 5 minutes or so. The rest of the time they will leave them in the nest and ignore them completely; this is a survival strategy to avoid drawing the attention of predators to the nest. Does with a new litter can take 24 hours to start lactating. Mismothering can be diagnosed if the kits have not been fed for 48 hours. Unfed kits will have thin abdomens and wrinkled skin due to dehydration.

**2 What are the common causes of failure of hand reared kits to thrive or survive?**
Hand rearing is difficult and time-consuming, especially if the kits are less than 7 days old. The most common causes of failure and death are aspiration pneumonia due to inhalation of milk into the lungs, and diarrhoea due to the failure to establish a normal gut flora. Death at around 4 weeks of age is also common due to intestinal *Escherichia coli* overgrowth.

**3 What housing and temperature is appropriate for hand rearing?** Kits under 7 days old will need to be kept at 27–30 °C. An incubator, heated hospital cage or the airing cupboard with thermometer can be used. Place the kits in a box lined with hay, maternal fur if available, or soft cloths/fleece bedding. The temperature can be lowered after 7 days if the kits are thriving.

## CASE 96

**What are the intramuscular injection sites in rabbits?** Intramuscular injection sites in the rabbit include the epaxial muscles (lying either side of the vertebral column in the lumbar region), the quadriceps muscle mass on the cranial aspect of the hindlimb (**96**), and the semimembranosus and semitendinosus muscles. The latter should be used with care as the sciatic nerve may be damaged with injection into this site. Large fluid volumes should be avoided (>0.5 ml) as well as irritant drugs, such as ketamine and enrofloxacin, as these may lead to tissue damage and muscle necrosis. Self-mutilation of the distal hindlimb has been reported following i/m injection and nerve damage in the rabbit. The authors' preferred site is the epaxial muscles, but care should be taken since a potential complication of any i/m injection is development of an injection abscess, which is difficult to treat at this site.

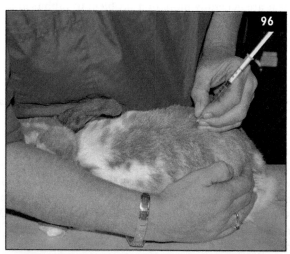

## CASE 97

**1 What procedure is being carried out (97)?** Indirect blood pressure (BP) measurement using a Doppler over the palmar common digital artery. The cuff width should be 40–60% of the circumference of the region it is to be placed around. In rabbits, placing the cuff just proximal to the elbow works well and minimizes patient stress. Providing sufficient coupling gel is applied to the palmar aspect of the distal limb, clipping of fur is not required. The cuff should be inflated above the expected systolic pressure to occlude the artery fully. As the cuff is slowly deflated, the first pressure wave through the artery should correspond to the systolic BP value. Normal systolic BP in the rabbit is 100–110 mmHg.

**2 What is the most likely reason for carrying out this procedure in a pet rabbit?** The most likely reason for carrying out this procedure is to assess cardiac output, which is directly related to BP. Blood pressure measurement is an important part of any cardiovascular examination, because hypertension can be a cause of heart disease and hypotension can be a sign of heart failure or severe hypovolaemia.

## CASE 98

**1 Which parameters are normal and which are abnormal?** A small amount of albumin is normal in adult rabbit urine and will give a weak positive for protein on urine dipsticks. This should be interpreted in conjunction with the SG. Very dilute urine that tests positive for protein is more likely to be significant. Although normal rabbit urine does not contain glucose, a slight glucosuria may occur with stress or hepatic lipidosis, and its occurrence should not be taken to indicate diabetes mellitus, which occurs very rarely in pet rabbits. Rabbit urine is normally alkaline, the pH ranging from 8–9, as is found in other herbivorous hindgut fermenters. It is essential to determine urine pH on fresh samples as the pH can be altered by bacterial contamination. Low urine pH in rabbits is usually related to catabolism due to anorexia or pyrexia. Rabbit urine should not normally contain ketones, and this is the most significant abnormality.

**2 What is the significance of these findings, and what is the likely reason for the rabbit's continued anorexia?** The original anorexia, due to oral pain, has given rise to a catabolic state with lipid metabolism, an associated hepatic lipidosis and the development of ketoacidosis.

## CASE 99

**What type of treatment is being carried out (99)?** The photograph shows an incubator unit set up for nebulization of a rabbit within an enclosed area. Nebulization has been described for the treatment of both upper and lower respiratory tract disease in rabbits. It may be used as a method of administration of mucolytic drugs, such as N-acetyl-cysteine, antibiotics and antifungal drugs directly into the respiratory tract. It also loosens secretions and aids nasal breathing. The medication (e.g. an antibiotic) is mixed with saline and administered via a nebulizer machine, usually twice daily for approximately 20 minutes. The rabbit is constrained within a small enclosed area. This method of drug administration involves minimal handling and stress to the animal. Proprietary nebulizers must produce droplets of <3 microns to penetrate to the lower respiratory tract.

## CASE 100

**What advice would you give this owner?** As a prey species, rabbits are likely to develop fear-related behaviours at times when they feel threatened or unable to flee from the threat. Aggression is often used as a last-ditch attempt to survive and, if successful, may be used more readily in the future. It is highly unlikely that this rabbit was exposed to regular handling by a variety of people when it was a young rabbit. Studies suggest that regular handling between the ages of 10 days and 6 weeks leads to less fearful rabbits. For a rabbit to exist as a cuddled pet, it really should be obtained when it is approximately 8 weeks old from a breeder who handles regularly from a young age.

Many attempts at handling are also inappropriate and an inexperienced person may increase the rabbit's apprehension. The owner should be advised to slowly build a relationship between the rabbit's favourite treat and stroking. With time and success this can progress to a lift on to the owner's lap and so on. Each time the rabbit is handled, attention must be given to protecting the rabbit's spine by keeping a hand under the rear end. The other hand can be placed over the shoulders or between the forelimbs.

It is unlikely that neutering will help to solve this problem, as this behaviour is not linked to the sex hormones.

## CASE 101

**1 Outline the aetiology of acquired dental disease?** Acquired dental disease is a progressive syndrome associated with changes in tooth structure, shape and occlusion. An exact aetiology is unclear, although it is likely to be multifactorial, involving the following:

- inadequate dental wear due to insufficient intake of coarse fibre in the diet
- nutritional deficiency, including calcium, vitamin D, vitamin A, magnesium and protein
- genetic predisposition – male Dwarf Lop rabbits seem to be particularly susceptible.

**2 Describe the progression of dental changes?** Lack of dietary abrasion of the cheek teeth leads to an excessive rate of eruption relative to the rate of wear. The increased occlusal pressure on the over-long exposed crowns (due to stretching of the masticatory muscles) resists further eruption. Tooth growth continues at the apex, leading to retrograde elongation of the reserve crowns, palpable as firm swellings on the ventral mandible. Apical intrusion damages germinal tissues, causing enamel dysplasia, and the incisors may develop transverse ridges. At this early stage there may be no clinical signs of dental disease.

The normal curvature of the cheek teeth crowns causes divergence from those of the opposing arcade as they elongate, reducing occlusal contact to only the buccal margins of the lower and lingual margins of the upper teeth. Consequently, uneven wear leads to the formation of sharp spurs on the opposite margins of the teeth, while the realignment of occlusal forces in a more lateral direction exacerbates the divergence and malocclusion as the tooth grows (acquired molariform malocclusion). Congenital molariform malocclusion is rare.

The excessive height of the molariform arcades prevents full closure of the mouth, thus separating the incisors, which elongate to compensate. Eventually they no longer occlude and overgrow (acquired incisor malocclusion).

Alveolar bone loss leads to loosening of cheek teeth and impaction of food material, causing further displacement and periodontal disease. Continued retrograde tooth elongation can eventually perforate the periosteum, with extension of any periodontal infection into the surrounding soft tissues.

The germinal tissue is gradually destroyed and, finally, tooth growth ceases.

## CASE 102

**1 What condition is illustrated?** The radiograph shows extensive ventral spondylosis, with exostoses involving lumbar vertebrae L1, 2 and 3. This is a common finding in older rabbits.

**2 What clinical signs may be associated with this condition, and how can the condition be treated?** Clinical signs include difficulty in grooming and an abnormal gait. The rabbit may also be incontinent and perineal urine scalding and caecotroph accumulation may be present. Treatment consists of improving hygiene, topical treatment of the perineum with antibacterial baths and barrier creams, systemic antibiotics as indicated for secondary bacterial infections and analgesics (e.g. NSAIDs, if renal function is normal). At best this condition can be managed and the rabbit's quality of life should always be considered. Euthanasia should be considered.

## CASE 103

**1 What other methods of individually identifying rabbits are used?** Pet rabbits may be identified by the placement of a microchip subcutaneously between the scapulae.

Leg rings are the most commonly used method of identification for show and exhibition rabbits in the UK, Australia, New Zealand and Japan. They should be placed above the hock of either hindlimb. Rabbits should be ringed at about 8–10 weeks of age, except in smaller breeds where earlier ringing is advisable. After this age it can be difficult to slide the ring over the hock joint. As the rabbit grows it is not possible to remove the ring without destroying it. Rings that are too small can cause restriction of blood supply, trauma and severe damage to the limb. Even appropriately sized and placed rings can cause problems if debris or fur builds up underneath them. In the UK, rings are available from the British Rabbit Council. They are available in ten sizes and allocated to specific breeds.

Other means of identification less commonly used are ear tags or studs and ear notching, and staining of the fur with dyes (temporary only as the dye will be lost with moulting).

**2 What method is required for exhibition purposes in the UK?** Leg rings are required for exhibition purposes in the UK. In the USA an ear tattoo is a requirement for entering a rabbit in a show.

## CASE 104

**1 What procedure is being shown (104)?** Placement of an intraosseous catheter in the proximal tibia.

**2 What anatomical sites may be used for this procedure?** Intraosseous catheters may be placed in the cranial edge of the tibial crest or in the trochanteric fossa of the proximal femur (104).

**3 Describe the technique.** The rabbit is anaesthetized and digital palpation is used to locate the femoral trochanteric fossa or the cranial edge of the proximal tibial crest. The area is shaved and then sterilized using a standard disinfectant. The area is covered with a sterile drape and sterile gloves should be worn. An 18–23 gauge, 2.5–3.75 cm (1–1.5 inch) needle is carefully inserted into the intramedullary cavity along the long axis of the bone using steady downward pressure. The needle should be flushed with sterile heparinized saline and a T-port or catheter bung attached. A light bandage is then placed over the catheter. Bone plugs can be avoided by using a spinal needle and stylet, or hypodermic needle with sterile surgical wire used as a stylet. Catheters are relatively well tolerated in the rabbit, although the leg may be bandaged to reduce limb movement and displacement of the catheter.

## CASE 105

**1 What are the advantages and disadvantages of using this method of fixation?** External fixators provide rigid stability and cause minimal soft tissue damage. They are often associated with shorter operative times and promote postoperative weight bearing. These implants eliminate the requirement for extensive bandaging, which can be difficult to maintain in many rabbits. One disadvantage is that some rabbits may self-traumatize the tissues around the fixator by excessive licking or chewing. This is a rare complication which is minimized by implementation of good perioperative analgesia and, in general, external fixators are well tolerated by rabbits.

**2 What factor influences the decision to use an open versus a closed surgical approach for placement of the fixator pins?** The basic principles of external fixator application in rabbits are similar to those for other species. If there is limited soft tissue covering the affected bone and the fracture is simple, it is advantageous to leave this tissue alone by approaching the surgery with a closed technique. With open fractures or comminuted injuries, debridement is often required. In these cases, an open technique is appropriate.

**3 What speed and angle are suitable for the placement of the pins?** The pins should be inserted at low rotational speed (150–300 revolutions per minute or rpm). High-speed drilling and manual insertion are not advised as both are associated with premature pin loosening. Ideally, the pins should be angled at approximately 70° to the longitudinal axis of the bone to minimize the risk of the pins pulling out. Positive-profile pins are available in small sizes and are preferred as they achieve a good level of purchase.

## CASE 106

**1 What is the expected lifespan of a pet rabbit?** Most pet rabbits can be expected to live for 5–8 years, but many may reach 10–12 years or more.

**2 What factors will affect lifespan?** Factors affecting lifespan include the following:

- *Breed* – smaller breeds tend to have a shorter lifespan.
- *Diet* – high-fibre, low-carbohydrate diets will maintain gastrointestinal and dental health and prevent obesity. High-fat diets are related to atherosclerosis and excessive vitamin D may lead to mineralization of blood vessels.
- *Husbandry* – housing, opportunity to exercise, stocking density, etc., will all affect the general health of the individual and the incidence of infectious disease.
- *Neutering* – early neutering of does will minimize the risk of developing uterine adenocarcinoma, a common cause of morbidity and mortality in does over 4 years of age.
- *Vaccination* against myxomatosis and rabbit haemorrhagic disease – will decrease the chance of mortality due to these infectious diseases.

3 **Is it possible to age a rabbit?** In general it is not possible to age a rabbit once adulthood is reached (6–8 months in most breeds). However, experienced owners and breeders may use various criteria. The claws do not generally project beyond the fur until maturity, and the ears feel 'tougher' in animals over 2–3 years than in younger animals whose ears are much softer. However, these factors are highly variable and no feature can be relied on. Deciduous dentition is shed at birth and permanent dentition is fully erupted from 3–5 weeks of age. Radiographic closure of the growth plates in rabbits occurs between 20 and 30 weeks (in the New Zealand White).

## CASE 107

1 **Which are the upper and which are the lower incisors?** The maxillary incisors have a markedly greater curvature compared with the mandibular incisors.

2 **Describe the extraction technique and postoperative care required.** The procedure takes place under general anaesthesia. Dental nerve blocks may also be used in conjunction. The aim is to break down the periodontal ligament to enable easy tooth removal. The appropriate end of a Crossley incisor luxator/elevator is gently inserted into the lateral and medial periodontal space and gradually worked under controlled pressure towards the apex of each tooth, carefully following the arch of the tooth. Movement of the instrument should be confined to the same plane as the tooth curvature to avoid fracture of the crown. Once loosened, a gentle rocking action is applied to the tooth until it lifts easily when gently pulled. Care must be taken not to twist the tooth, which may also lead to tooth fracture.

Before complete extraction, the tooth is pushed into the alveolus to crush the germinal tissue at the apex and prevent regrowth. The absence of pulp in the apex of the removed tooth suggests failure to destroy the germinal tissue completely, which should then be curetted by insertion of a bent sterile hypodermic needle into the alveolus. In all cases, prior to gaining consent, the owner should be advised of the possibility of tooth regrowth. This eventuality is most likely if the crown is fractured and the proximal fragment left *in situ*, requiring extraction once re-erupted.

Preoperative analgesia should be augmented and continued for 5–7 days post surgery, along with a course of systemic antibiotics (if clinically indicated) and gut motility stimulant drugs. The owner may need to assist the rabbit with grooming and to grate/chop hard foods.

3 **What additional considerations are there in cases of acquired incisor malocclusion?** In cases of acquired incisor malocclusion there are usually concurrent problems in the cheek teeth arcades that must also be addressed. Correction of cheek tooth elongation

may allow the incisors to be brought back into occlusion with only coronal reduction through burring, although the reduced curvature of lower incisors in advanced cases may make this impossible.

Extraction of incisors in cases of acquired malocclusion is technically more difficult, as the teeth may be brittle and possess longer or deformed reserve crowns. Roots may also become embedded in the socket due to periapical reaction. The presence of periodontal or periapical infection enhances the risk of postoperative abscessation. Preoperative radiography is essential to assess the whole dentition and may even negate the need to extract the incisors if apical changes suggest that growth has ceased.

## CASE 108

**1 Give the order, family, subfamily, genus and species of the domestic rabbit.** All domestic rabbits are descended from the European wild rabbit: order Lagomorpha, family Leporidae, subfamily Leporinae, genus *Oryctolagus*, species *Oryctolagus cuniculus*.

**2 How many chromosomes does the domestic rabbit possess?** The domestic rabbit has 22 pairs of chromosomes.

**3 To what genus do wild American rabbits belong?** Genus *Sylvilagus* (e.g. *Sylvilagus floridanus*, the Eastern Cottontail rabbit; *S. bachmani*, the Brush rabbit.

**4 Are Jack rabbits true rabbits?** Jack rabbits belong to the genus *Lepus* and are hares. They possess 24 pairs of chromosomes.

**5 Are Belgian hares true hares?** Belgian hares are a breed of rabbit (*Oryctolagus cuniculus*).

## CASE 109

**1 What injection technique is being shown (109)?** Intraperitoneal (i/p) injection.

**2 What are the potential complications associated with this procedure in the rabbit?** This injection technique is rarely necessary in pet rabbits and has been primarily described in laboratory rabbits. Good restraint is essential to avoid any sudden movements. Fluids should always be pre-warmed to body temperature. Care should be taken to avoid penetration of the bladder, especially if it is full. The thin-walled caecum may also be punctured with this technique as it lies in the right ventral abdomen. Intraperitoneal injections should always be made paramedian and caudal to the umbilicus to avoid the kidneys, liver and spleen. Always draw back to check the syringe contents prior to injection and stop and repeat the procedure if urine, blood or intestinal contents are aspirated.

## CASE 110

**1 How can you determine if this is indeed true diarrhoea?** True diarrhoea needs to be distinguished from uneaten caecotrophs or abnormally soft caecotrophs that adhere to the perineum. Relevant questioning during history taking can generally distinguish between the two situations. If there is true diarrhoea, no normal faecal pellets are passed. If this is caecotroph material, normal hard faecal pellets will still be passed or may be stuck among the adherent material. Rabbits with true diarrhoea are generally systemically unwell and deteriorating, with associated dehydration and abdominal pain. Caecotrophs have a characteristic strong 'vinegary' odour due to the volatile fatty acids present, and they are coated in mucus.

**2 If you determine that true diarrhoea is not present, what can cause this presentation?** Caecotrophs may remain uneaten or be abnormally soft for many reasons:

- Back or joint pain or restriction of movement (e.g. spondylosis, spondylitis, arthritis) so that the rabbit cannot bend to reach the anus and eat its caecotrophs.
- Obesity – the rabbit cannot physically reach its anus to eat the caecotrophs.
- Dental or other oral pain.
- Low-fibre, high-carbohydrate diets can predispose to abnormally soft caecotrophs.
- High-protein diets – may affect palatability of caecotrophs.
- Overfeeding leading to no calorific need for caecotroph ingestion.
- Lack of space and exercise.

## CASE 111

**What is your diagnosis, and how would you manage this case?** These are the signs of acute renal failure (ARF).

Acute renal failure (ARF) may be seen in older rabbits due to sudden filtration failure by the kidneys resulting in fluid deficits, acid–base and electrolyte imbalances and accumulation of uraemic toxins in the systemic circulation. Acute renal failure is potentially reversible, if diagnosed quickly and treated appropriately, but the prognosis remains guarded and full recovery can take several months. In contrast to chronic renal failure, affected rabbits with ARF usually present with non-specific symptoms such as anorexia, lethargy and depression and no loss of body condition. Secondary dehydration and gastrointestinal disturbances may also be seen. Urine production may be normal initially but can progress to oliguria. Azotaemia with concurrent isosthenuria or hyposthenuria is considered diagnostic. Animals that become oliguric may also develop hyperkalaemia and metabolic acidosis. Accurate anamnestic details may reveal evidence of exposure to nephrotoxins (e.g. aminoglycosides, sulfonamides, tetracyclines, lead batteries). Enlarged kidneys may be palpable on physical examination, and ultrasonography and/or radiography of the urinary tract is useful to confirm this finding and in the former case assess for any changes to renal architecture. A sterile urine sample should be submitted for urinalysis and culture to screen for infectious causes. Potentially nephrotoxic drugs should be discontinued and aggressive fluid therapy started to correct renal perfusion, replace fluid deficits, correct electrolyte and acid–base imbalances and reduce the azotaemia. Concurrent supportive therapy for any secondary gastrointestinal ileus and/or gastric ulceration is recommended. The volume of urine produced should be carefully monitored.

## CASE 112

**1 What is the most common leukocyte found in rabbit pus?** The predominant leukocyte found in the pus of rabbits is the neutrophil. In contrast to most mammalian species, rabbit neutrophils contain acidophilic granules and are easily confused with eosinophils.

**2 What is the bacterium most commonly isolated from rabbit pus?** Although classically the literature describes these cases as occurring secondary to infection with *Pasteurella multocida* (a Gram-negative bacterium), other microorganisms, particularly *Staphylococcus aureus* (a Gram-positive bacterium), are commonly implicated. Therefore, it should not be assumed that any condition producing pus in pet rabbits is caused by *Pasteurella*: culture and sensitivity are necessary in these cases.

## CASE 113

**1 What do the abnormalities marked with an asterisk indicate?** While there is no absolute leukocytosis, there is a relative neutrophilia (92%) and leukopenia (6%). This is often seen in acute inflammatory responses such as acute bacterial infections. The elevated TP, albumin, RBC count and PCV indicate dehydration. The increased glucose is likely due to stress-induced endogenous steroid release, since true diabetes mellitus is rare in pet rabbits. Elevated AST, ALT and ALP are likely due to anorexia and catabolism.

**2 What is the likely diagnosis?** This animal had a clostridial enterotoxaemia. This is common in recently weaned rabbits. Sudden diet change and stress are further predisposing factors.

## CASE 114

**1 What levels of dietary fibre, fat and protein are appropriate for adult pet rabbits (114)?** Adult pet rabbits should be offered a diet high in fibre (with total dietary fibre levels in the range 20–25% with indigestible fibre >12.5%). Fat should be restricted to approximately 2.5% of the diet and moderate amounts of good quality protein (12–16%) are appropriate.

**2 How do the nutritional requirements of lactating does and growing juveniles differ from those of non-breeding adults?** Lactating does require a diet with a higher fat (3%) and protein content (18–19%) than their non-breeding counterparts. During lactation, energy requirements will increase to 3–4 times maintenance needs and therefore the quantity of food offered must be increased accordingly.

Similarly, a protein level of 15–16% and a fat level of 3% are conducive for growth in weaning rabbits.

For both of these groups, fibre remains the single most important dietary component and it is important not to compromise fibre levels in order to increase the fat and protein content of their diet. Some manufacturers produce highly palatable pelleted foods that encourage greater energy intake but in doing so these may provide an insufficient level of indigestible fibre. Fibre levels should not fall below 16% for growing or breeding rabbits.

## CASE 115

**1 What is the condition, and how is it related to the teeth?** The rabbit has epiphora, which has caused a secondary superficial pyoderma and local alopecia below the eye. In acquired dental disease, inadequate dental wear leads to excessive exposed crown length and consequent increased occlusal pressure. This in turn resists further eruption, so that tooth growth continues in a retrograde direction. In the case of the first maxillary incisor, this can impinge on the nasolacrimal duct, which runs close to the apex of the incisor, causing a partial or complete obstruction. Secondary

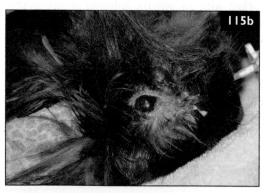

bacterial infection of the duct often follows (dacryocystitis), where milky fluid can be expressed from the lacrimal sac by gentle pressure below the medial canthus (115b). In more advanced dental disease, root elongation or a periapical abscess of the first maxillary premolar may also block the duct.

2 **What other indicators of dental disease might be apparent on routine physical examination, even before inspecting the oral cavity?** Apical elongation of the lower cheek teeth can be appreciated as irregularities in the ventral margin of the mandible. Maxillary masses may also be palpable. Decreased lateral movement of the mandible may be present on gentle manipulation, due to elongation and abnormal curvature of the cheek teeth and spur formation.

Uneven molariform wear due to malocclusion forms sharp spurs that lacerate the buccal and lingual mucosa. The pain associated with these lesions stimulates salivation and interferes with swallowing, resulting in ptyalism. This is seen as a wet or matted chin, brisket or forelimbs, perhaps with secondary dermatitis. Inability to groom results in poor coat condition and may make existing ectoparasite infestations more severe (e.g. *Cheyletiella parasitivorax*). Pain may also prevent caecotrophy, with consequent accumulation of caecotrophs around the anus. (There may also be a reduced appetite for caecotrophs with inappropriate diets.) This malodorous mass is often misinterpreted as diarrhoea by the owner, and it predisposes the animal to fly strike. Perineal skin may become inflamed, particularly if the passage of urine is impeded.

The rabbit may be currently anorexic (perhaps with gut stasis) and reluctant to drink from a dropper bottle, or the owner may report a history of periods of anorexia as successions of lesions heal, only to reform once mastication resumes. This is reflected in a gradual net loss of body condition.

Buccal lesions may become infected and give rise to facial abscesses. Continued retrograde tooth elongation eventually results in perforation of the periosteum and extension of periodontal infection to form periapical abscesses. Those arising from maxillary cheek teeth may be associated with exophthalmus (molars), intrusion into the nasal passages, causing rhinitis and respiratory noise (PM1), or swelling below the medial canthus (PM2, PM3).

## CASE 116

1 **Is this suitable accommodation?** This hutch is far too small as sole accommodation for a rabbit. It does not give any opportunity for exercise or for the rabbit to exhibit all normal behaviours, including grazing. There is a serious welfare issue in keeping a rabbit in this manner.

2 **What advice would you give an owner on the minimum size of a hutch?** Due to the large variety in size of domestic rabbits, definitive hutch sizes are difficult to give. A good rule to use is that the hutch must allow the rabbit easily to sit upright on its hindlimbs with its ears erect, to stretch out fully and to perform three consecutive hops in the same direction. In addition, an exercise area, preferably on grass, must be provided for at least several hours a day.

## CASE 117

**What are the potential complications associated with this technique?** Rabbits tolerate nasogastric tubes well and placement is as described for the cat. Rabbits are obligate nasal breathers with extremely sensitive nasal mucosa and may therefore strongly resent tube placement. In these cases sedation or general anaesthesia may be necessary. In non-fractious or moribund cases, use a local anaesthetic gel to lubricate a 5–8 FG radiopaque feeding tube or apply local anaesthetic ocular drops to the nasal opening. Measure the length required, using the nasogastric tube, from the nares to the last rib. Elevate the head and insert the tube into the ventral nasal meatus, aiming ventrally and medially. Flexion of the head when the tube is at the level of the larynx will help ensure that it passes down the proximal oesophagus rather than the trachea. Rabbits do not always cough if the tube is placed in the trachea; therefore, the placement of the tube should be checked radiographically. Attach tape with butterfly wings to the tube and glue it to the fur on the head or, alternatively, suture the tube in place. An Elizabethan collar may be required in some animals. Care should be taken to flush the tube after each feed with water and, because the tube can easily become blocked, only dilute syringe feeding formulas should be used. The nasogastric tube may be left in place for several days, until the animal starts to eat on its own. Once recovered, the rabbit will eat despite the tube being *in situ*.

Potential complications associated with nasogastric intubation include inadvertent placement of the tube into the trachea and iatrogenic damage to the nasal mucosa, with associated epistaxis and secondary bacterial sinusitis. Great care should be taken when applying this technique to dyspnoeic rabbits as it may cause a worsening of the dyspnoea since the tube partly occludes one nostril and rabbits are obligate nasal breathers.

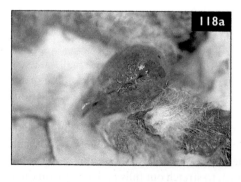

## CASE 118

**What are the commonly observed post-castration complications in rabbits, and how may these be avoided?** Haemorrhage; swelling; wound breakdown; wound infection; scrotal haematoma (**118a**) and seroma formation; penile prolapse (**118b**). A closed technique should always be used in rabbits to prevent postoperative herniation of abdominal contents. Excessive swelling and haemorrhage may be avoided by overnight hospitalization of the rabbit, since most cases are a direct result of overactivity or sexual activity in the immediate postoperative period. Self-trauma or loosening of the ligatures may also result in haemorrhage. The risk of self-trauma can be minimized by leaving the prescrotal incision open, similar to castration techniques in cats. This avoids the use of sutures which may cause irritation or local reaction. Infection may be avoided by good aseptic operating technique. Adequate analgesia and prokinetics in the postoperative period and close observation will also help to reduce the potential for complications.

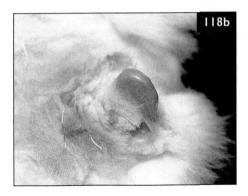

## CASE 119

**1 What is the procedure being performed (119a, b)?** The photographs show a rabbit receiving an i/v blood transfusion into the marginal ear vein. The donor rabbit should weigh at least 1 kg and cross-matching is not required at the first transfusion. Up to 1% of body weight can be safely collected from the donor. Use the jugular vein and commercially prepared collection and storage bags. If only a small blood volume is being collected, use a 10 ml syringe containing 1.2 ml citrate phosphate dextrose adenine. Heparin (5–20 units/ml of blood) can also be used as an anticoagulant. An in-line filter should be used for administration. The blood may be given directly to the recipient via the marginal ear vein as a slow i/v bolus in an emergency but ideally an in-line filter should be used. Blood should be replaced at 6–12 ml/kg/h. Blood groups have been identified in rabbits, but initial transfusion reactions are rare. Respiration and heart rate should be monitored for evidence of a transfusion reaction.

**2 For what conditions is this procedure indicated?** Blood transfusions are indicated in cases of severe anaemia where the haematocrit has dropped below 0.1–0.15 l/l (10–15%), depending on the duration of anaemia and clinical signs. There are many different causes of anaemia in the rabbit and these can be divided into two categories: regenerative and non-regenerative. The two main causes of a regenerative anaemia are haemorrhage (internal and external) and intravascular haemolysis. Haemorrhage may be caused by trauma, flea bites, intestinal bleeding, splenic haemorrhage, hepatic haemorrhage, uterine adenocarcinoma and uterine endometrial venous aneurysm. Intravascular haemolysis is rare in rabbits and could potentially be caused by *Mycoplasma haemofelis* infection, lead toxicity and immune-mediated disease such as autoimmune haemolytic anaemia, which has been described in laboratory rabbits associated with lymphosarcoma. Non-regenerative anaemia occurs in rabbits secondary to chronic infections (e.g. dental abscesses), chronic renal failure, neoplasia (e.g. lymphoma) and toxins.

## CASE 120

**What are the standard radiographic views used for imaging in the rabbit (120)?**
Standard radiographic views are as for the cat and dog; however, in addition, skull radiographs (lateral, dorsoventral, left and right 20–30° oblique and rostrocaudal views) should also be taken to assess for evidence of dental disease. For the lateral thoracic view, the forelimbs should be drawn forward as far as possible to minimize superimposition over the cranial lung fields.

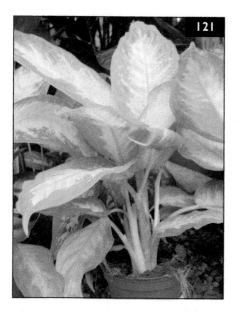

## CASE 121

**What plants are known to cause toxicity in rabbits?** There are few documented cases of plant toxicity in rabbits. Instead, rabbits are relatively resistant to plants that cause toxicity in other species (e.g. ragwort, comfrey, laburnum and deadly nightshade). The houseplant *Dieffenbacchia* (**121**) is poisonous to rabbits if ingested, as are avocado plant leaves. All plants grown from bulbs (e.g. crocuses, daffodils and lilies) are toxic to rabbits. Common garden plants that may be toxic to pet rabbits include anemones, arum, bindweed, foxgloves, oak leaves, poppies, speedwell, lupins, primroses, privet, rhododendron, wisteria and yew. Although not native to the UK, *Amaranthus* spp. (e.g. 'pigweed') may cause ascites in rabbits if ingested. It is possible that this plant could occur on wasteland sites. In the USA, woolly pod milkweed (*Asclepias eriocarpa*) can cause paralysis of the neck and incoordination if eaten, a condition known as 'head down disease'. This plant does not grow in the UK.

## CASE 122

**What auxiliary test could be used for the *in vivo* diagnosis of active Encephalitozoonosis in this case, alongside measurement of antibody titres?**
Measurement of serum C-reactive protein (CRP) levels.

In vivo diagnosis of *Encephalitozoon cuniculi* infection is challenging because clinically healthy domestic rabbits often have high antibody titres (IgG) and seroconversion may be indicative of acute, subclinical infection or simple exposure. A concurrent positive IgM titre may help in evaluation of the infective status of the affected rabbit as it is indicative of active infection. Encouraging results derive from evaluation of adjunct diagnostic tests which may aid in the diagnosis. Analysis of specific acute phase proteins (APPs) circulating in the blood where they modulate the innate immune system's response to tissue injury has given promising results. APPs are generally produced following tissue injury and prior to inflammation, as part of the acute phase response (APR) which occurs before a specific immune response. APPs are therefore one of the first indicators of a pathologic process. CRP is a positive APP (it increases in response to tissue injury) which, in dogs, modulates the efficiency of some inflammatory cells, thereby modulating the immune system during inflammation. Recently, rabbits suspected of having *E. cuniculi* infection were found to have significantly elevated levels of CRP compared to a healthy control group. CRP levels in rabbits not infected by *E. cuniculi* averaged less than 10 mg/l, whereas CRP levels were in the range of 30–200 mg/l in rabbits suspected of *E. cuniculi* infection. CRP is known to increase within 24 hours of an inflammatory insult and appears to be a major APP in rabbits.

## CASE 123
How would you optimize analgesia during the immediate postoperative period and ensure that an adequate level of analgesia is maintained throughout? Analgesia provided postoperatively depends on the anaesthetic technique utilized. Commonly used methods include the use of oral or parenteral medications such as non-steroidal and opioid drugs.

However, depending on the frequency of administration, there will be occasions when the animal may suffer additional pain prior to the next dose being administered. In these cases using a continuous rate infusion is a useful technique to keep the level of analgesia constant. Agents such as dexmedetomidine, ketamine and methadone can be used in combination. Loading doses are given intravenously, followed by a constant rate infusion. These infusions can be given alongside fluid therapy and are often used pre-emptively prior to surgery. Standard regimes employed often mirror those used in other species and are being increasingly utilized in rabbits.

Suggested dose rates are as follows:

| Agent | Loading dose (mg/kg) | Infusion rate (mg/kg/h) |
| --- | --- | --- |
| Ketamine | 0.5 | 1.2 |
| Dexmedetomidine | 0.0005 | 0.0003 |
| Methadone | 0.5 | 0.1 |

It is also important to consider the benefits of other analgesics alongside these, such as using local anaesthetic blockades and non-steroidal drugs. Once the CRI is no longer required, parenteral use of alternative opioid drugs is often continued, with buprenorphine being in common use due to its longer duration of action.

## CASE 124

**1 Identify the indicated mite and eggs.** The mite shown is *Cheyletiella parasitovorax*. The most common mites seen in rabbits are the fur mites *Cheyletiella parasitovorax* and *Leporacarus gibbus* (formerly *Listrophorus gibbus*), and the ear mite *Psoroptes cuniculi*. Other mites occasionally seen on rabbits are *Demodex cuniculi*, *Notoedres cati*, *Neotrombicula autumnalis*, *Psorobia lagomorphae*, *Dermanyssus gallinae* and *Sarcoptes* spp.

**2 What are the identifying features?** *C. parasitovorax* is a non-burrowing mite; it causes seborrhoea, alopecia and pruritus. Adult mites are large and have hook-like accessory mouthparts. *L. gibbus* is also a non-burrowing mite. Adult females of this species are sometimes described as similar to a flea in appearance, with a striated cuticle, dark, sclerotic head and short legs with no clasping adaptations. Membranous flaps arising from the first set of legs attach the mites to a hair. Males have a long adanal process and adanal suckers. *P. cuniculi* may be found causing skin lesions. These mites are large – up to 0.07 mm in length – and may be seen with the naked eye. They have an oval body shape, pointed mouthparts and three jointed pedicles with funnel-shaped suckers.

**3 Which related organism is not generally associated with seborrhoea?** *L. gibbus*. Clinical signs are alopecia, pruritus and sometimes a moist dermatitis. Many cases are asymptomatic, but hypersensitivity reactions to this mite are reported in rabbits.

## CASE 125

**What common conditions can be diagnosed on ultrasonographic examination of the urogenital tract in the female rabbit?** Ultrasonography is an extremely useful tool in the investigation of urogenital disease in the rabbit. Uterine hyperplasia, endometrial polyps, pyometra, uterine adenocarcinoma, hydronephrosis, renal cysts, renoliths, ureteral calculi and hydroureter may all be diagnosed using this technique. The renal cortex, medulla and pelvis may be evaluated for any abnormalities. The ovaries may also be evaluated. Differentiation between cystic calculi and hypercalciuria is possible in addition to bladder evaluation and measurement of bladder wall thickness. Ultrasound-guided needle biopsy or aspirate may be performed under sedation, including cystocentesis for sterile urine samples. A full caecum (common in the latter part of the day) may impede examination, as may intestinal ileus.

## CASE 126

**1 What problems can be caused in rabbits by lack of early socialization?** Lack of socialization with humans will increase fearfulness and stress in young rabbits when they do interact with people. This can lead to behavioural problems such as fear-related aggression. Increased stress levels will have effects on gastrointestinal motility, especially at the sensitive time of weaning when normal gut flora is becoming established, and this can be a factor in the incidence of weaning associated enteritis, mucoid enteropathy or gut stasis in older rabbits.

**2 How can these problems be prevented?** Studies suggest that gentle handling from as young as 10 days of age has a positive effect on the rabbit's ease of approaching both familiar and unfamiliar people. Female rabbits handled early in life have also been shown to have better breeding performance, possibly because they are less stressed. Breeders should aim to handle kits for a few minutes once or twice a day from about a week old. They should stroke the doe first to ensure their hands are covered in her smell, in order to prevent maternal rejection.

## CASE 127

**What preoperative and intraoperative considerations are essential in rabbits undergoing a surgical procedure?** Prior to anaesthesia, stress should be kept to a minimum. The rabbit should be clinically evaluated to assess for any pre-existing disease which could affect its response to the anaesthetic and this should be addressed. Perioperative analgesia should be instigated for painful procedures. Because they are unable to vomit, rabbits should not be starved prior to general anaesthesia. Anorexic animals should be given nutritional support and fluid therapy to avoid hepatic lipidosis and dehydration. Rabbit skin is thin and tears easily and the dense fur may block the clipper blades, making clipping of the fur difficult. Blades should be sharpened and cleaned regularly to ease the process, and the skin should be spread flat with the clipper close to the skin when clipping commences. Aseptic preparation of the surgical site is routine; however, excessive use of alcohol-based preparations should be avoided to prevent chilling and hypothermia. A patent airway should be maintained throughout the procedure and oxygen supplied at all times. Intravenous access should be maintained via an indwelling intravenous cannula and fluid therapy provided via this route. During surgery the rabbit should be placed on a heat mat or heated operating table and the body temperature closely monitored. Alternatively, circulating warm-water blankets or forced-air warmers may be used. In rabbits the eyes protrude laterally from the orbit. Ocular lubricants should be applied to the eyes during anaesthesia to prevent drying of the cornea and exposure keratitis (**127b**). Correct positioning during surgery is imperative, since respiration is significantly

171

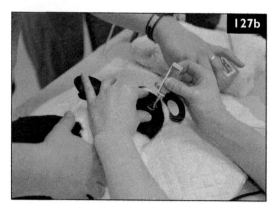

127b

impeded if the animal is placed in dorsal recumbency. The weight of the abdominal viscera presses on the diaphragm, particularly in large or obese rabbits. To avoid this, the head and thorax should be elevated. Subclinical respiratory disease may also be present, which can compromise respiration further.

## CASE 128

**1 What potential sources of vitamin D are available to rabbits?** Vitamin D precursors are synthesized in the skin following exposure to natural sunlight. The vitamin is also present in sun-dried hay and is incorporated into most concentrate rations. For optimum levels it is recommended that rabbits obtain their vitamin D from all three sources. Exposure to sunlight has additional psychological and physiological benefits for many rabbits.

**2 A reduced intestinal absorption of which mineral is likely to result from a chronic vitamin D deficiency in rabbits?** Vitamin D deficiency results in reduced intestinal absorption of phosphorus and can therefore lead to hypophosphataemia and osteomalacia.

Unlike other mammals, rabbits do not require vitamin D for intestinal calcium absorption unless dietary calcium levels are low.

**3 How might vitamin D toxicity present?** Vitamin D toxicity in rabbits can result in soft tissue mineralization, especially in the kidneys and aorta.

## CASE 129

**A lateral abdominal radiograph from a rabbit is shown. What normal anatomical features can be seen?** Normal abdominal contents that may be easily visualized include the simple stomach, intestines (duodenum, long caecum with appendix, large intestine), kidneys, liver and bladder. Food and caecal pellets are always present in the stomach. The caecum lies on the right side of the abdomen. Rabbits often have large amounts of retroperitoneal fat, which displaces the kidney ventrally. In intact female rabbits the uterus may be visible situated ventral to the large intestine and dorsal to the bladder. The bladder may normally contain a small number of calcium carbonate crystals, which will appear radiodense, as is evident in this radiograph.

## CASE 130

**1 What procedure is being carried out?** Computed tomography (CT) is being carried out on an anaesthetized rabbit. The technique requires the animal to be anaesthetized or suitably contained so that it will not move and placed within a rotating X-ray beam. It is the diagnostic imaging technique of choice for evaluation of the head, vertebral column and all calcified structures. It is also useful in visualizing air-filled structures such as the ear canal and tympanic bullae. It is less useful for differentiating soft tissue structures unless an intravenous contrast agent is used to highlight well-vascularized areas.

**2 For what conditions is this indicated in the rabbit?** CT is extremely useful in the diagnosis of upper respiratory (e.g. rhinitis/sinusitis, apical dental infection, foreign body, neoplasia) and lower respiratory tract disease, dental disease, vestibular disease associated with otitis media/interna, facial and ear base abscesses and conditions affecting the spinal vertebrae A diagnosis is often made where more conventional imaging techniques have not been successful. CT imaging often shows up more extensive soft tissue and bony changes associated with facial abscesses in the rabbit than are immediately apparent radiographically. This is helpful in determining prognosis and appropriate surgical treatment. Access to CT imaging is becoming increasingly available to vets in practice and is an extremely useful diagnostic tool.

## CASE 131

**List the differential diagnoses for infectious causes of diarrhoea in rabbits of this age.**

- Coccidiosisis is very common in young rabbits. There are at least 16 species of *Eimeria* reported to occur in rabbits. For example, *Eimeria magna*, *E. flavescens*, *E. piriformis* and *E. intestinalis* can all cause intestinal coccidiosis. Mixed infections often occur, sometimes in conjunction with other pathogens such as *Escherichia coli*. Diarrhoea is also a symptom of hepatic coccidiosis caused by *E. steidae*. Affected animals may also have ascites and hepatomegaly and can be icteric.
- *Cryptosporidium parvum* has been described in rabbits, but it is not a major cause of disease.
- *Giardia duodenalis* can cause catarrhal enteritis rarely in rabbits.
- Colibacillosis. *E. coli* is not a normal inhabitant of the rabbit GI tract and pathogenic strains can cause severe enteritis.
- Salmonellosis. *Salmonella typhimurium* and *S. enteriditis* are the most common isolates.
- Tyzzer's disease. *Clostridium piliforme* causes a typhlitis, enteritis, hepatitis and myocarditis.

- Clostridial enterotoxaemia. Overgrowth of intestinal *Clostridium spiriforme* (and occasionally *C. perfringens* and *C. difficile*) is precipitated by stress, low-fibre high-carbohydrate diet, and high levels of pathogen in the environment in intensive situations.
- Other bacterial infections that can cause diarrhoea are *Klebsiella pneumoniae, K. oxytoca, Lawsonia intracellularis* and *Pseudomonas aeruginosa*.
- Rotavirus. Concurrent infection with *E. coli* increases the severity of clinical signs.
- Coronavirus. Rabbit enteric coronavirus has been associated with diarrhoea in rabbits and it can also cause pleural effusion and cardiomyopathy.

## CASE 132

**1 What procedure is depicted?** Cannulation of the nasolacrimal duct. Rabbits possess a single lacrimal punctum situated towards the medial canthus in the lower palpebrum. For cannulation a topical ophthalmic local anaesthetic is first administered into the eye. Excellent illumination is required for the procedure. The rabbit is restrained and a lacrimal cannula or intravenous catheter sleeve carefully introduced into the punctum. The nasolacrimal duct may then be flushed with saline solution to clear debris or with topical medications such as antibiotics. Gentle pressure should only be applied while flushing as there is a risk of iatrogenic rupture of the lacrimal sac if the duct is blocked.

**2 In what circumstances is this procedure indicated?** This procedure is indicated in cases of chronic conjunctivitis, where the lacrimal punctum fills with purulent material, or in cases of dacryocystitis, which often occurs secondary to spread of infection from the nasal cavity or to blockage of the duct by elongated tooth roots, especially the maxillary incisors. In these cases, radiography of the skull is indicated, including contrast studies of the nasolacrimal duct.

## CASE 133

**1 What is your diagnosis based on this photograph?** Renal calculus. Urolithiasis is the term generally used to indicate the presence of calculi within the urinary tract. Calculi may be present in the kidneys, as in this case.

**2 What are the most likely causes of this condition in pet rabbits?** The cause is likely to be multifactorial, and diet, anatomy and infections may all play a role. Rabbits have an unusual calcium metabolism, with an efficient and vitamin D3-independent absorption mechanism of dietary calcium. Serum total calcium levels directly reflect the dietary intake and any excess calcium is mainly excreted via the kidneys as calcium carbonate. Urine is therefore the major route of calcium excretion in rabbits (45–60% of calcium is excreted by this route compared to

2% in other mammals). The excreted calcium precipitates in the alkaline urine forming calcium crystals and giving normal rabbit's urine a thick, creamy consistency. The rabbit's kidneys are paired retroperitoneal organs situated in the posterior part of the abdomen on each side of the vertebral column. They have a relatively primitive structure as they are unipapillate (one papilla and one calyx enter the ureter directly) compared to the multipapillate kidneys of most mammals.

**3 How would you manage this case?** Treatment of urolithiasis depends on the location of the stones and the severity of the lesions. The location of the calculus should be accurately determined by radiography and/or ultrasonography prior to attempting any procedure to remove it. Nephrectomy may be indicated if a calculus in the renal pelvis is causing urine flow obstruction and irreversible damage to the renal parenchyma. Nephrotomy can be an alternative treatment option when the function of the affected kidney is still adequate (based on laboratory results, ultrasonography and excretory urography) and the renal parenchymal damage is minimal. Dietary changes are important as part of the treatment and prevention plan. Measures should be taken to promote exercise, reduce obesity and monitor water intake. Supportive care and appropriate antibiotic treatment should be provided as required.

## CASE 134

**1 What is the normal rectal temperature range in a rabbit?** Normal rabbit rectal temperature is 38.5–40.0 °C.

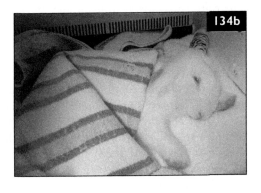

**2 At what body temperature in a rabbit would you start to be concerned about the risk of hypothermia?** Rectal temperatures below 38.5 °C should demand one's attention and, where possible, the cause should be identified and addressed.

**3 What strategies would you employ to maintain normothermia?** Heating strategies should be put into action if the temperature drops steadily, and these include heating devices such as:

- 'hot hands' (warm water in examination gloves)
- an incubator (**134b**)
- forced heated air blankets
- microwavable heat pads

## CASE 135

**1 Name the structures 1, 2, 3, 4 and 5.**
1 = Ascending colon; 2 = ileum; 3 = ileocaecal tonsil; 4 = caecum; 5 = vermiform appendix.

**2 Describe the movement of ingesta through these portions of the GI system.**
As ingesta in the ileum approaches the ileocaecocolic junction, it is directed towards the proximal ascending colon and is mixed and separated into two portions, liquid and solid ingesta. Indigestible lignified material accumulates in the lumen, while the digestible fraction (including complex carbohydrates, plant proteins, digestive enzymes, soluble ions and intestinal secretions) settles near the circumference of the proximal colonic haustra. The digestible particles along with fluid are sent retrograde by reverse peristaltic action into the caecum. Meanwhile, through a series of coordinated contractions of the intestinal wall, the indigestible particles are directed into the descending colon where absorption of water and electrolytes takes place. This material is eventually passed from the anus as hard faecal pellets, the production of which coincides with feeding activity. Typically, a 2.5 kg rabbit will produce on average 150 faecal pellets each day. Caecal contents undergo microbial fermentation, producing volatile fatty acids, proteins and amino acids. Periodically, the production of hard faeces is halted and caecal contents are passed back into the proximal colon. Here they form mucus-encapsulated pellets, which are moved very rapidly into the descending colon and are passed as caecotrophs. These are eaten directly from the anus by the rabbit. This process follows a marked circadian rhythm.

## CASE 136

**1 Describe the procedure for collection of cerebrospinal fluid in the rabbit.** CSF may be collected in small volumes from both the cisterna magna (atlanto-occipital approach) and the lumbosacral epidural space (lumbar approach) in rabbits. Samples are collected under general anaesthesia with the rabbit intubated. The area is shaved and surgically prepared prior to the procedure. Sterile drapes and gloves are used. For collection from the cisterna magna, the rabbit is placed in lateral recumbency and the neck flexed towards the sternum. A 22 gauge 3.75 cm (1.5 inch) spinal needle is inserted at right angles to the vertebral column in the dorsal midline at a point equidistant from the cranial margins of the wings of the atlas and 2 mm caudal to the occipital protuberance (136) arrow. The needle is slowly advanced towards the nose, until a slight 'pop' is felt on penetration of the dura and subarachnoid membranes. The stylet is removed and CSF should gather in the hub of the needle. Do not aspirate; allow the CSF to drip into a plastic container (glass causes leukocytes to stick to the walls of the container). A maximum volume of 0.5 ml only should be collected. Analyse immediately or refrigerate the sample. For the lumbosacral tap, the position is similar to that in the dog with the epidural space 0.75–2.5 cm (0.3–1.0 inch) below the skin surface.

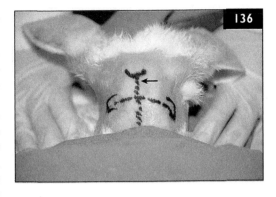

**2 What are the conditions in which this procedure is indicated?** This procedure is indicated in cases of neurological disease to collect samples for cytology and culture, for example to help diagnose listerial infections. Polymerase chain reaction (PCR) analysis for *E.cuniculi* may also be performed on cerebrospinal fluid (CSF) samples.

## CASE 137

**1 What are your differential diagnoses for urine scalding in rabbits?** Differential diagnosis for urine scald include: cystitis, hypercalciuria/urolithiasis, *Encephalitozoon cuniculi*, renal failure, obesity, posterior paralysis and ectopic ureter.

**2 What initial diagnostic tests would be advisable to perform?** Urine specific gravity, urine protein:creatinine ratio, urine dipstick analysis, serum biochemistry blood profile – particularly urea and creatinine (**137a**).

**3 Describe two ways you could obtain a sterile urine sample from this animal.** A sterile urine sample may be obtained using cystocentesis or via placement of a urinary catheter.

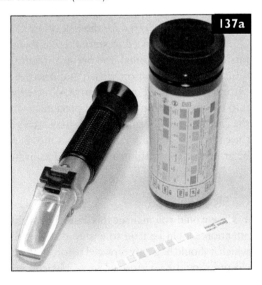

The technique for cystocentesis (**137b**) is similar to that used in felines. Collection of urine can be performed under sedation or conscious, depending on the nature of the rabbit. If cystocentesis is performed conscious, a local anaesthetic cream (e.g. EMLA) can be applied on the skin 15–20 minutes prior to the procedure to desensitize the skin to the needle.

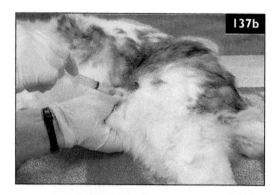

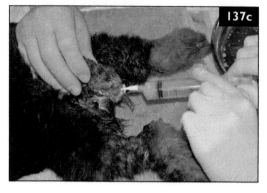

An assistant restrains the rabbit with the spine supported and hindlimbs gently stretched backwards. The antepubic region is clipped and aseptically prepared. A small gauge needle (23–25 gauge) attached to a 5–10 ml syringe is required to aspirate the urine. Ultrasonography may be used to locate the bladder if it is not immediately obvious on palpation.

Placement of a urinary catheter is readily performed in doe rabbits (**137c**). General anaesthesia or heavy sedation is required. Premedication with a benzodiazepine drug is recommended. (Midazolam is routinely used by the authors, combined with buprenorphine.) Dipyrone/hyoscine (Buscopan®) can also be used concurrently at 0.1–0.25 ml/kg s/c to reduce the risk of urethral spasm.

The patient is placed in sternal recumbency with a rolled-up towel or sandbag raising the hips. If soiled, the perineal region should be carefully washed in warm dilute antiseptic solution, rinsed and dried. A sterile lubricated urinary 3–5F gauge catheter is advanced into the vulva, directed ventrally along the floor of the vagina into the urethal ostium. Correct placement is confirmed by the presence of urine in the catheter. Small urine volumes may sometimes be obtained by misplacement of the catheter in the vaginal vestibule. Once in place, a three-way tap and syringe can be attached to control urine flow and aspirate a sample for analysis.

## CASE 138

**1 How would you manage this case?** The visible herniated organ is the bladder. Close attention should be paid to ensure that the bladder has not been traumatized, after which it should be gently replaced before the wound is reclosed. A three-layer abdominal closure should be performed in rabbits comprising intramuscular, subcutaneous and intradermal sutures. Rabbits commonly chew skin sutures so placement of these should be avoided. Elizabethan collars may be used in rabbits displaying self-trauma, but these are not used routinely as they are stressful to the rabbit and prevent caecotrophy.

**2 What are your differential diagnoses for the midline swellings post spay procedure?** Differential diagnosis for a swelling around a recent abdominal surgical site include a postoperative seroma or haematoma, infection, suture material reaction or herniation of abdominal contents following wound dehiscence or incomplete linea alba closure.

**3 How would you determine if a case requires corrective surgery?** Differentiation of the aetiology will involve clinical examination of the patient, possibly assisted by ultrasonography to determine the composition of the contents of the swelling. Seromas and haematomas often resolve spontaneously over a period of time. Suture material reactions can be present, particularly if catgut has been used. Close monitoring for wound dehiscence is required along with monitoring for clinical signs associated with intra-abdominal adhesions.

If infection is present, it is preferable to explore surgically to obtain samples for culture and to debride necrotic material. Herniation is often easy to diagnose, with many hernias reducible under palpation. If herniation has occurred, surgical correction is required.

## CASE 139

**1 What are the objectives of any rabbit dental treatment?**
The objectives are to:
- correct the length and occlusal surface angle of the incisors
- reduce the height of the molariform arcades to a level appropriate to the normal
- remove any spurs
- establish a normal plane of molariform occlusion, allowing a normal range of masticatory movement, with wear evenly distributed across the entire occlusal surface.

**2 What technique can be used for dental correction?** Dental correction is best achieved by grinding the teeth with high- or low-speed rotating burr, performed under general anaesthesia with a mouth gag and cheek dilators (**139b**). Soft tissue damage and thermal injury to the tooth pulp can be avoided with the use of tongue depressors to shield and retract

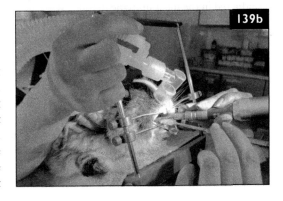

139b

tissues and the application of water periodically to the tooth to dissipate heat. Excessive shortening of the cheek teeth should be avoided, as mastication of fibrous food is prevented if the arcades are taken out of occlusion, predisposing to postoperative anorexia, gut stasis and, potentially, hepatic lipidosis. There is frequently elongation of pulp tissue in affected teeth and exposure of this due to overzealous shortening will result in pulp exposure and pain. In advanced dental disease there is also the chance that tooth growth may cease before occlusion is regained.

3 **Do dental rasps have a place in rabbit dental procedures?** The use of dental rasps for coronal reduction is outdated and contraindicated. The force required when rasping can weaken the periodontal ligament, causing the tooth to loosen which in turn increases the periodontal space. This may predispose to the development of dental infections.

4 **What is the likely prognosis for this rabbit?** In early cases, dentistry and an improved diet may be curative. However, changes in shape, position and direction of growth of teeth are permanent and lead to malocclusion.

Maloccluded growing teeth will generally always require periodic correctional dentals. Nevertheless, provision of a suitable diet will slow the progression and help prevent nutritional deficiency, which in turn will support the integrity of dental tissues and guard against periodontal infection. Ultimately, tooth growth may cease. In the absence of spurs or infection, and with provision of an appropriate diet, the rabbit may manage even with only a few remaining teeth.

## CASE 140

**What alternative methods of euthanasia could be used?** Administration of an injectable sedative or anaesthetic prior to euthanasia would be recommended in this case. Inhalation anaesthetic should not be used as a sole agent as the rabbit is likely to struggle, vocalize and demonstrate apnoea in response to the noxious gas.

Once the rabbit is sedated or anaesthetized via s/c or i/m route, intracardiac or intrarenal injection of barbiturate can be performed. Euthanasia should always be conducted in the most humane manner, with the patient's welfare a primary concern.

## CASE 141

1 **What procedure is being carried out on this cadaver (141)?** Collection of a bone marrow sample by needle aspiration from the proximal femur.

2 **Describe how this is performed on a live rabbit.** This procedure should be carried out under general anaesthesia under aseptic conditions. Potential sites for bone marrow collection include the femur, humerus, pelvis and proximal tibia.

- The area over the collection site is clipped and surgically prepared.
- Overlying soft tissue structures and the periosteum are infiltrated with 2% lidocaine. Opiate analgesia should also be provided.

- Sample collection by aspiration is favoured due to the small bones and relatively thin cortices. A needle and stylet is introduced with a drilling action into the medullary cavity.
- The stylet is removed and a 5 ml syringe is attached with 1 ml sterile phosphate-buffered saline with 0.24% EDTA.
- 0.5 ml of marrow is aspirated. The needle should be repositioned if nothing is aspirated at first. Few complications have been reported following this technique in the rabbit, with mild haemorrhage being the most common.
- Core biopsy is also possible if care is taken, using the same technique but with a 3.75 cm (1.5 inch) 18 gauge needle.

**3 For what conditions is this procedure indicated?** Aspirates are used to look at cell morphology and myeloid:erythroid ratios. Core biopsies should be used to evaluate hypocellular marrow. The most common indications for bone marrow examination in the rabbit are anaemia, thrombocytopenia, leucopenia and, less commonly, neoplasia (lymphosarcoma), infectious disease (*Pasteurella multocida, Staphylococcus aureus*) and bone marrow dysplasia.

# CASE 142

**1 What age group does this disease primarily affect?** As a general rule, ERE affects young farmed rabbits between the ages of 6 and 14 weeks, but odd cases have been reported in older animals in commercial establishments.

**2 What are the associated clinical signs?** The most characteristic clinical signs are abdominal distension and mild watery diarrhoea. In some cases there may be increased borborygmi and passage of mucus from the rectum. In addition, many affected rabbits show non-specific signs of illness, including inappetence and lethargy. The mortality rate is high.

**3 How is the disease diagnosed?** As the aetiological agent in unknown, a diagnosis can usually be made based on the clinical pattern and postmortem (PM) findings in an outbreak of weanling mortality. On PM, typically there is pronounced abdominal distension due to dilatation of all segments of the GI tract, including the stomach. The intestinal and stomach contents include gas, liquid and sometimes mucus. Macroscopic congestive or inflammatory lesions (as seen in cases of coccidiosis, clostridial disease or colibacillosis) are typically absent.

**4 Which antimicrobial drugs have been shown to be of some benefit in reducing mortality rates or preventing outbreaks of the disease?** Tiamulin, bacitracin, tylosin (alone or in combination with apramycin) and some coccidiostats have been shown to have some effect in controlling the disease. The effectiveness of these drugs is likely related to controlling the development of secondary infections, which would add further complications to the rabbit's immune status. The aetiological agent has yet to be identified and, as is often the case

181

with other infectious diseases of farmed rabbits, control measures should not rely entirely on medicinal therapy. Farm management practices, nutritional therapy and improved hygiene and sanitation are important considerations.

## CASE 143

**1 What are your differential diagnoses?** Differential diagnoses for seizures in rabbits are shown in the table:

| Parasitic aetiology | Infectious aetiology | Toxic aetiology |
|---|---|---|
| Encephalitozoonosis | Listeriosis | Lead toxicity |
| *Baylisascaris procyonis* infestation (cerebrospinal nematodiasis) | Bacterial encephalitis/ meningitis | Ingestion of plant toxins, rodenticides |
| Toxoplasmosis | Bacterial abscess | and herbicides |
| Sarcocystis | | |
| **Other** | | |
| Heat stroke | | |
| End-stage disease (e.g. viral haemorrhagic disease, liver failure, septicaemia, renal failure, intestinal obstruction and ileus) | | |
| Pregnancy toxaemia | | |
| Hypoxia | | |
| Neoplasia | | |
| Metabolic disease (renal failure, liver failure), | | |
| Electrolyte abnormalities | | |
| Epilepsy (especially in rabbits with white fur and blue eyes) | | |
| Cardiovascular disease (e.g. arteriosclerosis) | | |

**2 What further diagnostic tests would you perform?** A complete history should be obtained to rule out access to potential toxins. Further diagnostic tests should include: a full neurological assessment of the animal, blood sampling for biochemistry and haematology to rule out metabolic disease and electrolyte disturbances and to look for evidence of inflammation or infection, full body and skull radiographs, cerebrospinal fluid tap, serology for *Encephalitozoon cuniculi* infection, blood heavy metal profile, and a CT or magnetic resonance imaging (MRI) scan.

**3 What are the treatment options?** Treatment options are symptomatic and are similar to those in other species. Diazepam or midazolam (by s/c, i/m or i/v injection or *per rectum*) can be given to control seizure activity. The dose rate for administration of diazepam during status epilepticus is 0.5 mg/kg i/v, repeated every 10 minutes up to three times as required. Rectal diazepam may be provided for the owner to administer in case of seizure activity in the home environment.

If no causative agent is identified, oral phenobarbital at 1–2 mg/kg/day can be started to try to control seizure numbers. Systemic antibiotics or specific treatments such as CaEDTA for lead toxicity or fenbendazole for *E. cuniculi* infection should be administered where appropriate. Supportive care with GI motility modifiers and syringe feeding critical care formula should also be given to address the anorexia.

## CASE 144

**1 What is the most likely diagnosis?** Antibiotic-associated diarrhoea and enterotoxaemia. In rabbits, antibiotics can alter the intestinal flora, leading to bacterial overgrowth of pathogenic species such as *Clostridium* spp. Amoxicillin-clavulanate is a high-risk antibiotic when given via any route and is contraindicated in rabbits.

**2 What is the prognosis?** The prognosis in this case is extremely poor. *Clostridium* spp. multiply, resulting in enterotoxaemia, dehydration, electrolyte loss and acute death. Prompt aggressive treatment is required.

**3 What are the treatment options?** Intravenous fluid therapy is required, along with nutritional support. The rabbit should be kept warm and the body temperature monitored. Cholestyramine is an ion-exchange resin that absorbs enterotoxins and may be useful if given early on. Probiotics can be administered orally. Metronidazole may be administered to act against anaerobic *Clostridium* spp. Analgesics may be indicated.

## CASE 145

An indoor rabbit has been seen eating the leaves of one of the owner's houseplants (145). The owner is concerned that this may be toxic to the rabbit, although no adverse clinical signs have been noted. **What is your advice?** This is a common problem in house rabbits; the owner may not always know the plant species. Ideally, the plant should be identified to allow further research to be carried out, although rabbits are relatively resistant to plant toxins. They are often not affected by plants that are highly toxic to other animal species (e.g. ragwort and deadly nightshade). The toxic side effects will depend on the amount eaten, the part of the plant ingested and the frequency of ingestion. In general, if no side effects are seen 6 hours post ingestion, it is unlikely that the animal will be affected.

General advice should be removal of the plant from the animal's reach and close observation of the animal over the next 24 hours. If GI side effects are seen, the animal should be given supportive care with fluid therapy, probiotics and intestinal stimulant drugs.

## CASE 146

**1 What condition is seen in this radiograph?** Widespread gaseous distension of the intestines indicates that non-obstructive ileus is present.

**2 What factors can affect gut motility?** Control of GI motility is complex. Motility is under the influence of the autonomic nervous system, prostaglandins and other hormones such as motilin. Autonomic nervous control is coordinated by the fusus coli ('pacemaker' of the gut) in the colon. Motilin, which enhances motility, is inhibited by high-carbohydrate diets. However, it is largely stimulated and maintained by a high throughput of non-digestible fibre (lignocellulose). Factors leading to decreased motility include: lack of dietary fibre; high dietary carbohydrate; anorexia; chronic dehydration; sudden change of diet; environmental stressors (e.g. proximity of predators, proximity of a dominant/competitive rabbit, change/destabilization of group hierarchy, change of housing, transport, extremes of weather/temperature, loss of a companion); pain; post-surgical adhesions; ingestion of toxins (e.g. lead); foreign body.

**3 What treatment would you initiate?** Treatment should consist of the following:

- *Fluid therapy* – to maintain the circulation and to rehydrate GI contents. In mild cases, s/c and oral fluids may be all that is required, but in more severe cases intravenous fluids are indicated. Maintenance volumes are 100 ml/kg/day.
- *Analgesia* – buprenorphine (0.01–0.05 mg/kg s/c or i/v q8h), butorphanol (0.1–0.5 mg/kg s/c or i/v q2–4h), carprofen (2–4 mg/kg s/c or i/v q24h), meloxicam (0.3–0.6 mg/kg s/c q24h or p/o q12h).
- *Gastrointestinal stimulants* – metoclopramide (0.5 mg/kg s/c q12h), cisapride (0.5 mg/kg p/o q12h) and ranitidine (4 mg/kg p/o q12h).
- *Assisted feeding* – commercially available high-fibre herbivore recovery diets. Always offer hay.
- *Exercise* – helps to stimulate GI motility.

## CASE 147

**1 What information, relevant to the dentition, can be gained from radiography?** The length and position of reserve crowns; growth status of the teeth; the patency of the nasolacrimal duct (contrast studies); bone changes due to osteomyelitis; bone density and quality.

**2 What standard views should be obtained?** Lateral, dorsoventral, rostrocaudal and lateral oblique views should be taken. Open mouth views may be useful in some cases.

**3 Describe the radiographic features of acquired dental disease, with reference to any abnormalities in the picture.** Once the exposed crowns have elongated to an extent that occlusal pressure resists further eruption, retrograde growth occurs. This is accommodated by remodelling of the surrounding jaw bone. With time, the tooth apex impinges on the cortex, seen as thinning of the incisive bone by the first upper incisor, and/or the ventral mandible by the lower cheek teeth. Eventually, the ventral margin of the mandible is deformed.

As a rule of thumb, the apices of the maxillary molariforms should not rise above the level of the arch of the primary incisors (a tangent taken parallel to the incisive bone) on the lateral view, suggesting excessive elongation of these teeth in the case shown.

Apical intrusion can result in distorted retrograde growth that deviates from the curvature of the tooth, following the topography of the supporting bone until finally perforating the periosteum.

If an abscess forms, a mixture of bone lysis and proliferation gives a mottled appearance typical of rabbit osteomyelitis. Occasionally, tooth growth continues around the abscess, producing bizarre forms.

The normal 'zigzag' occlusion of the opposing molariform arcades is gradually lost.

## CASE 148

**An owner asks about deworming her pet rabbit. What is your advice?** Rabbits do not need to be routinely wormed, as endoparasites are rarely pathogenic in this species. The rabbit pinworm, *Passalurus ambiguus*, is commonly found but does not cause clinical signs even in relatively large numbers. *P. ambiguus* ova may be easily detected on faecal microscopy (148a) and adult worms are common incidental findings on postmortem examination of caecal contents (148b).

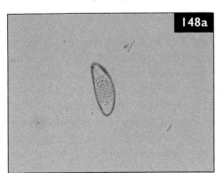
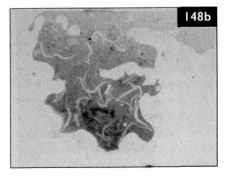

Cestodes species (e.g. *Taenia*) may be problematic if rabbits are allowed to graze on contaminated pastures. Prevention of cestode infection is achievable by limiting access to definitive host (e.g. dog, cat, fox) faecal matter with environmental hygiene.

Faecal analysis should be performed if an endoparasite problem is suspected, and treatment given only if a pathogenic infection is diagnosed.

## CASE 149

**1 What is the normal rectal temperature of a rabbit?** The normal rectal temperature of a rabbit is 38.5–40.0 °C.

**2 What methods can be used to warm a hypothermic rabbit patient, and how is this achieved?** The first stage in treating a hypothermic rabbit is to prevent further heat loss by wrapping the animal in insulating material such as bubblewrap, foil or blankets. Warmed i/v fluids should be instigated immediately. The rabbit should then be slowly warmed to its optimal body temperature (**149**). Methods for warming patients include the use of hospital cages, incubators and brooders, heaters and fans to maintain room temperature, hot water bottles, 'hot hands' and microwave-heated plastic or grain bags, hairdryers, water circulating heat mats, warm air blanket systems and electric heat pads. Rectal temperature should be recorded regularly, as should the immediate environmental temperature of the patient.

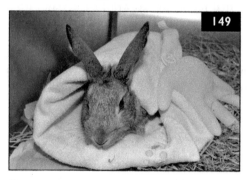

## CASE 150

A domestic rabbit is presented with weight loss and polydipsia, and you are suspicious of renal disease. **How would you collect a urine sample (150), and what simple adjunct test could be performed on this sample to evaluate renal function?** Urinalysis has to be part of a basic diagnostic work-up in cases where urinary tract disease is suspected. A free-catch urine sample can yield useful information, but ideally the sample should be collected in a sterile manner. Cystocentesis is better performed under ultrasonographic guidance with sedation in most cases. Alternatively, catheterization of the urethra is easily performed in both male and female anaesthetized rabbits.

Urine specific gravity (SG) 1.003–1.036 is considered normal in the rabbit and therefore evaluation of the ability of the kidneys to concentrate or dilute urine can be valuable, if combined with serum urea and creatinine measurement, to distinguish between pre-renal, renal and post-renal azotemia. Traditional clinical pathology indicators of nephrotoxicity such as serum urea, serum creatinine and urinalysis parameters (including total protein, albumin and sediment examination) are considered relatively insensitive and non-specific indicators of modest renal dysfunction, as changes in these biomarkers tend to occur only after extensive damage has been sustained by the kidneys. Damage of at least 65% to 75% of the nephrons is necessary before a significant increase in serum creatinine is observed and changes in routine urine analysis can be detected. In these cases, proteinuria seems to occur earlier than biochemical changes, although protein levels need to be evaluated along with urine specific gravity and sediment because healthy rabbits may have trace proteinuria. Measuring urinary protein:creatinine ratio (a UPC ratio of 0.11–0.47 is reported to be normal in rabbits) may be a useful test in clinical practice, alongside urine specific gravity, to quantify the proteinuria. Persistent proteinuria, in urine with inactive sediment, is an indication of renal tubular or glomerular disease and can be used as a marker of the severity of renal disease, to monitor disease progression and as an important prognostic factor.

## CASE 151

**1 What toxin is likely to be involved?** Fungicides belonging to the triazine group may cause toxicity in rabbits.

**2 What treatment is indicated?** Treatment is symptomatic, with supportive care and fluid therapy. The rabbit should be admitted to hospital and access to the toxin stopped. Start i/v fluid therapy with lactated Ringers solution and syringe feeding (50 ml/kg p/o 3–5 times a day) with a commercial critical care formula for rabbits. Probiotics and intestinal stimulant drugs such as ranitidine (4 mg/kg s/c or p/o q8–12 hours) metoclopramide (0.5 mg/kg s/c q6–8h) may be useful. If the rectal temperature is low (normal values 38.5–40 °C), provision of a heat mat or placement in an incubator is indicated. If the rabbit appears in abdominal discomfort, analgesia should be provided (e.g. buprenorphine, 0.05 mg/kg s/c q6–8h).

**3 What is the prognosis?** Prognosis is good with appropriate supportive care.

## CASE 152

**1 What skeletal injuries are rabbits prone to if they are handled incorrectly?** Spinal fracture, spinal luxation, usually at L6/L7.

**2 List the factors that make them susceptible to these injuries.** Long, curved spine; powerful, well-muscled hindlimbs, which are kicked strongly backwards in attempts to escape; naturally lightweight skeleton (8% bodyweight compared with 12–14% in most other mammals of comparable size); osteoporosis due to inactivity or metabolic bone disease will increase risk of injury; selective breeding of meat breeds (e.g. New Zealand White) for rapid growth.

## CASE 153

**1 What is your diagnosis?** Encephalitozoonosis. The photograph shows Gram-positive protozoal parasites within macrophages. *Encephalitozoon cuniculi* is an obligate intracellular protozoal parasite, belonging to the order Microsporidia.

**2 How is this disease transmitted?** In pet rabbits the most likely route of infection is via ingestion of spores from urine-contaminated food and water. Transplacental infection and infection via the respiratory route following inhalation have also been reported. The parasite infects the host cell and eventually the host cell ruptures, releasing parasitic spores, which go on to infect other cells. The life cycle lasts 3–5 weeks. Rupture of the host cell causes inflammation and results in clinical signs in the host animal.

## CASE 154

**What are the indicated structures on the rapid Romanovsky-type (Rapid-Diff) stained blood smear from a 3-year-old female French Lop rabbit (154)?** Normal rabbit thrombocytes (platelets).

## CASE 155

**1 What are your differential diagnoses?** Head tilt is usually a sign of vestibular dysfunction. Differential diagnoses for head tilt in the rabbit include: central nervous system (CNS) disease (cerebellum or medulla oblongata) such as bacterial infection, toxicities, encephalitozoonosis, *Baylisascaris procyonis* infestation (cerebrospinal nematodiasis) in the USA, toxoplasmosis, rabies (not UK), herpesvirus, degeneration, cerebrovascular accidents or neoplasia; peripheral nervous system disease (vestibular labyrinth or cranial nerve (CN) VIII) such as otitis media/interna, head trauma, iatrogenic ear cleaning and possibly 'idiopathic vestibular syndrome', although this has yet to be categorized in rabbits. Otitis media/interna in rabbits is usually associated with bacterial infection such as *Pasteurella multocida*, although other bacteria are often involved.

**2 What further diagnostic tests are indicated?** A full clinical examination with neurological assessment is indicated. This is essential to differentiate between peripheral nervous system disease and CNS disease. Rabbits with CNS disease are likely to present with further clinical signs such as tremors or hypermetria. Peripheral nervous system disease usually involves the vestibular labyrinth or vestibular nerve (CN VIII). Full haematology should be performed to rule out the possibility of an infection.

Radiography under sedation can be performed, but radiographic changes are often only visible in chronic cases. In advanced cases, dorsoventral and lateral oblique radiographic views of the skull may show increased bone density and thickening of the tympanic bulla or complete destruction of bone. CT is the gold standard diagnostic test for ear disease.

MRI is useful for identifying abnormalities of the brain and spinal cord, however the lengthy general anaesthetic time required for the scan, along with limited availability results in MRI not being commonly performed in rabbits.

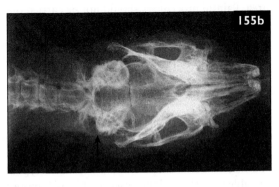

In this case, radiography of the tympanic bullae revealed severe bilateral changes, with chronic wall thickening associated with otitis media, and, on the right side, destruction of the craniolateral bulla wall (shown with arrow in 155b).

**3 What treatment options are there, and what is the long-term prognosis in this case?** Treatment options for otitis media/interna and vestibular disease in rabbits consist of long-term antibiotic administration based on culture and sensitivity results, topical administration of ear preparations (e.g. enrofloxacin drops) and NSAIDs. Initially, nursing care is indicated with nutritional support and syringe feeding. Animals should be housed on paper or soft towels and furniture should be kept to a minimum to prevent self-trauma secondary to circling or rolling.

In severe cases the external ear canal should be flushed under general anaesthesia with endoscopic guidance using copious amounts of warm sterile saline with suction. Bulla osteotomy may be indicated if CT indicates infection within the middle ear. Removing pus may help alleviate pressure.

Long-term prognosis is variable. Although the head tilt is unlikely to resolve fully, improvement of clinical signs is seen in many cases. Rabbits adapt and learn to cope with a head tilt and can go on to have a good quality of life.

## CASE 156

**1 What restraint technique is being used in this rabbit (156) and how is it achieved?** Hypnotization, trancing or tonic immobility. The rabbit is tipped or rolled gently on to its back while being held firmly to prevent kicking. The ventrum can be gently stroked in the direction of the fur as the grip is slowly and quietly released. Most rabbits will remain on their backs in an apparently trance-like state. There may be initial twitching of the limbs. A loud noise or sudden movement will end the 'trance' and the rabbit will jump up.

**2 What procedures may be carried out using this technique?** Ideally, this technique should not be used for restraint. When it is utilized, the rabbit should be in the position for only a short amount of time to facilitate a non-painful procedure such as examination of the ventrum, clipping nails or clipping fur around the perineal area. Painful procedures should not be carried out using this method of restraint.

**3 What response is believed to underlie this behaviour?** This behaviour is believed to be a fear response, with the rabbit 'playing dead' in response to being manipulated by a predator. To be maintained in this position for long periods of time is thought to be highly stressful for a rabbit.

## CASE 157

**1 What is the likelihood of diabetes mellitus occurring in a pet rabbit?** Diabetes mellitus is rarely seen in rabbits, but it has been reported in New Zealand White rabbits, where it is similar to maturity-onset (type 2) diabetes in humans. Herbivores are able to withstand the absence of insulin more readily than carnivores, and they are therefore less susceptible to developing diabetes.

**2 How would you diagnose this condition?** Diagnosis is based on blood parameters (repeated raised blood glucose levels over 13.9 mmol/l, increased plasma triglycerides and significantly elevated glycosylated Hb concentrations), glycosuria and clinical signs (polyuria and polydipsia). Normal values for the i/v glucose tolerance test in rabbits have been developed; however, this test is used to identify mild cases that will rarely require insulin therapy and it may therefore be unnecessary. Normal blood glucose levels in rabbits range from 4.2–8.3 mmol/l. It should be remembered that these levels may be elevated secondary to stress, shock, transport or handling.

If diabetes is suspected, the patient should be hospitalized and blood glucose concentrations should be checked in a non-stressful environment. Glycosuria is also non-diagnostic for this condition in rabbits, as it too may occur following stress, periods of anorexia secondary to hepatic lipidosis, and ketosis. These conditions are more common and should be ruled out first. Ideally, the owner should obtain a urine sample in the rabbit's normal environment to rule out stress factors. Normal fructosamine values have yet to be evaluated in rabbits, although work has been published with values from both clinically ill and healthy rabbits. The significance of fructosamine levels in the rabbit is therefore uncertain.

**3 What treatment would you commence in the event of diabetes mellitus being confirmed?** Insulin therapy may not be necessary, because diabetes in rabbits responds well to an increase in dietary fibre intake and a reduction in weight in obese individuals. Initial supportive care may, however, be necessary in this individual, consisting of syringe feeding a high-fibre critical care diet until the animal is self-feeding and stimulation of intestinal motility using metoclopramide (0.5 mg/kg s/c q6–8h).

## CASE 158

**1 What is the likely underlying condition?** Fur pulling in entire female rabbits, without a history of contact with an entire male, is likely to be associated with pseudopregnancy.

**2 What other clinical signs may be associated with this problem in does?** Other clinical signs that may be present include mammary gland hyperplasia, with or without secretion of milk, nest building and increased aggression. The condition lasts for approximately 16–18 days, during which time the doe will not let herself be mounted. Mammary hyperplasia may lead to mastitis. If prolonged or recurrent, this condition may develop into hydrometra or pyometra. The doe will create a nest from bedding materials and insulate it with a lining of plucked fur.

**3 Why does this condition occur in the rabbit?** Pseudopregnancy in does occurs as a direct result of normal elevations in plasma prolactin concentration post ovulation. This may occur following a sterile or unsuccessful mating (rabbits are induced ovulators) or following ovulation stimulated by mounting of another doe.

**4 What are the treatment options available?** No treatment is required, as this condition is usually self-limiting. Ovariohysterectomy is indicated for long-term prevention. In chronic cases the use of cabergoline (5 µg/kg q24h for 4–6 days) has been anecdotally reported as being effective in the treatment of persistent lactation in does. (NB: This drug is not licensed in rabbits and its side effects and therapeutic actions are not known.)

## CASE 159

**1 What is this condition?** Splay leg. This developmental problem occurs in young rabbits from a few days of age to a few months of age. Affected animals present with an inability to adduct one or more limbs. The hindlimbs are more commonly involved than the forelimbs. The rabbit may be severely lame or have a clumsy gait.

Radiographic examination may detect skeletal deformities, including femoral neck anteversion, femoral shaft torsion and coxofemoral luxation/subluxation.

**2 What is the prognosis?** The prognosis is poor. Full limb function is unlikely and euthanasia is usually indicated.

3 **What advice should be given to the owner?** The owner should be advised that this is an inherited simple autosomal recessive condition and therefore the affected animal should not be used for breeding. Breeding again from the parents should also be discouraged.

## CASE 160

1 **How would you restrain a rabbit in order to take a jugular blood sample?** The rabbit should be positioned on the edge of the table, with an assistant holding the head up (**160**). The neck should be extended so that the nose points vertically upwards. The forelimbs should be gently extended and allowed to rest over the edge of the table. A towel can be used to 'burrito' the rabbit to keep the spine and hind limbs secured.

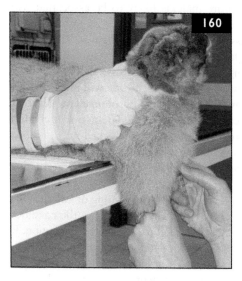

2 **What are the risks of improper restraint?** Improper restraint can lead to injury to both the rabbit and the handler.

When positioning the head, the neck should always be extended to prevent kinking the trachea, which would impede respiration. As rabbits are obligate nasal breathers, the nares must not be inadvertently occluded, as this will cause the rabbit to panic.

Towel wrapping is useful to secure the hindlimbs and spine, reducing the risk of struggling and kicking, which could cause fractures or luxation of the spine.

## CASE 161

1 **What type of cast is shown?** A cellular cast.
2 **Which type of cast, seen in dogs and cats, is almost never seen in rabbits, and why?** Hyaline casts are almost never seen in rabbits. These consist of predominately protein precipitates caused by a renal proteinurea, and they dissolve in alkaline rabbit urine. Cellular and granular casts consist of conglomerates of white blood cells or sloughed renal tubular epithelium cells with mucoproteins. These are less likely to be found in aged rabbit urine samples, as the effect of alkaline urine on the mucoproteins may lead to cast disintegration. Cystocentesis and rapid in-house examination of urine sediment are useful in detecting casts in rabbit urine.

3 **What is the significance of finding casts in rabbit urine?** The presence of casts in urine indicates renal damage. Casts may be one of the first detectable clinical pathology changes in renal disease.

## CASE 162

1 **What are the possible causes of death in this animal?** Differential diagnoses for sudden death with haemorrhage include:

- viral haemorrhagic disease (VHD) – sudden death with bleeding from the nose and mouth is a characteristic sign of this calicivirus infection
- trauma – from a predator, or self-trauma to head (e.g. from being startled)
- anticoagulant rodenticide poisoning (e.g. warfarin).

2 **What postmortem findings would confirm your diagnosis?** Postmortem findings with VHD are of a necrotizing hepatitis and splenitis. The liver is pale, enlarged and friable and has a lobular pattern. Lung haemorrhage and a frothy, bloody exudate are found in the trachea, nasal passages and mouth. Widespread disseminated intravascular coagulation (DIC) causes fibrinous thrombi and haemorrhage in most organs, especially the lungs, heart and kidneys. Histopathologically, acute hepatic necrosis, acute nephropathy and the DIC and haemorrhage are confirmed. Diagnosis can be confirmed by haemagglutination and enzyme-linked immunosorbent assay (ELISA) tests and detection of the calicivirus by electron microscopy.

Trauma would be apparent on postmortem examination of the carcass, and there would be an absence of signs of other disease. Bruising or wounds would be visible.

Rodenticide poisoning is a less likely cause of death. Anticoagulants such as warfarin, coumachlor and indandione derivatives interfere with prothrombin production in the liver and cause multiple haemorrhages throughout the musculature, especially over bony prominences, and internal haemorrhages including epistaxis. External haematomas may also be present.

## CASE 163

1 **What indications are there for the use of corticosteroids in rabbits?** Corticosteroids should be used sparingly in rabbits. They are occasionally required for their anti-inflammatory properties, but even small one-off doses may cause pathological changes in rabbits. The use of corticosteroids in the treatment of neoplastic conditions and allergic and autoimmune disease has not been well documented.

2 **What side effects may be seen when treating rabbits with corticosteroid drugs?** There is little information concerning corticosteroid efficacy in pet rabbits, although side effects have been well documented in rabbits used for research. These include a reduction in wound healing and significant immunosuppression.

Immunosuppression can make the rabbit more susceptible to infections such as *Pasteurella multocida* or to precipitation of overt disease secondary to subclinical or latent infections. Hepatic disease and diabetes may also occur. Due to side effects potentially leading to debilitating disease and even death, corticosteroids should be used in rabbits with extreme care.

## CASE 164

**1 What are the clinical signs associated with *Encephalitozoon cuniculi* infection in rabbits?** Clinical signs of *E.cuniculi* can include head tilt, torticollis, hindlimb paresis, paralysis, retarded growth, collapse, tremors, convulsions, urinary incontinence, renal failure, cataracts and lens-induced uveitis, death.

**2 What diagnostic tests are available for confirming *E. cuniculi*?** Serum antibody assay tests are most widely used for diagnosis of this disease. Immunofluorescent assays, ELISA assays and carbon immunoassays have also been used.

Postmortem examination with histopathology of the kidneys or brain can provide a positive diagnosis. Granulomatous changes or the organisms themselves are detected in tissues. Stains used for histopathology include Giemsa, carbolfuschin or Gram's stain (Gram positive).

Other diagnostic tests that are less commonly used include culture of spores from urine or examination of centrifuged urine samples for spores using modified trichrome stains or immunofluorescence.

**3 What are the potential difficulties in reaching a definite diagnosis of active disease?** A major problem with this disease is the difficulty diagnosing an active infection in live rabbits.

Postmortem examination is the only definitive diagnosis for this parasite, with typical lesions seen in the kidney and/or brain. ELISA tests are used at present in the UK to measure serum antibody levels to the parasite. Measurement of antibody titres is used, with rising levels of antibodies indicating an active infection. A positive antibody response on its own indicates previous exposure to the parasite. It does not, however, distinguish between early infection, active infection, chronic asymptomatic infection or previous exposure and recovery. Infection in rabbits may be asymptomatic, with carrier status occurring. To differentiate between these, a rising antibody titre over a period of time would need to be demonstrated.

## CASE 165

**1 What zoonotic organisms may be transmitted from rabbits?** Potential zoonotic organisms include: *Trichophyton mentagrophytes*, *Microsporum* spp., *Cheyletiella parasitovorax*, *Encephalitozoon cuniculi* (unlikely – immunosupressed individuals potentially at risk), rabies virus (not UK), *Franciscella tularensis* (not UK), lymphocytic choriomeningitis virus (unlikely), *Pasteurella multocida* (unlikely), *Haemodipsus ventricosus* (vector for tularaemia), *Pneumocystis carinii* (immunosuppressed individuals only at risk), *Salmonella* spp., *Yersinia pseudotuberculosis*, *Leptospira* spp. (unlikely), *Giardia* spp. (uncommon).

**2 What other health risk may rabbit owners face?** Other health risks include allergy to rabbits. It is estimated that 11–15% of owners and vets are allergic to rabbits and/or rodents. Dander and aerosolized urine proteins are the suspected antigens. Reactions include runny eyes and nose, coughing, wheezing and skin lesions such as urticaria and eczema, and this can develop into serious anaphylaxis. Hypersensitivity can develop over weeks and years and is more likely if other allergies exist and if familial predisposition exists. Different types of allergic reaction are involved. Type I (immediate) hypersensitivity is initiated by interaction of mast cells and basophils and release of chemical mediators such as histamine, serotonin and heparin. These act as messengers that target eosinophils, platelets, monocytes and T-lymphocytes. The final reaction is smooth muscle contraction, vascular dilatation and increased vascular permeability. Type IV hypersensitivity (cell-mediated allergic reaction) is caused by antigens reacting with sensitized T-lymphocytes (e.g. allergic contact dermatitis).

## CASE 166

A 5-year-old female French Lop rabbit has signs of urine scald of the perineum (166a). On clinical examination an excessive skin fold is observed surrounding the perineum. Describe both the medical and surgical treatment options in this case. This condition is often seen secondary to obesity in pet rabbits and some resolution of clinical signs may occur with weight reduction and increased exercise. Most skin infections can be treated with daily bathing using diluted chlorhexidine, although

it is imperative to rinse and dry the area afterwards. Antibiotics may also be necessary.

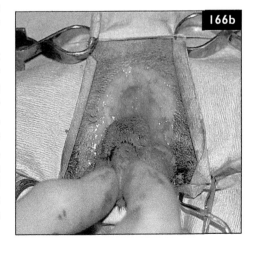

The flap of excess skin will collect soft faeces and deviate the normal flow of urination. This will predispose the rabbit to urine scalding, myiasis (fly strike) and localized skin infections. Some animals will continue to have problems, despite weight loss. These animals may benefit from dermoplasty, where a C-shaped section of skin is excised cranial to the genital opening, so removing the skin flap (166b).

## CASE 167

An owner brings a 4-month-old rabbit to the veterinary practice for vaccination (167). What preventive health care topics should you discuss with the owner at this stage? Topics to discuss with a new owner include the importance of diet, vaccination, neutering, husbandry, companionship, space requirement, environmental enrichment, handling techniques, fly-strike prevention and insurance.

## CASE 168

**1 Describe the abnormality shown in the radiograph (168a).** The radiograph reveals a comminuted, articular fracture of the proximal tibia and fibula. In combination with the physical examination findings, radiography confirms that the fracture is closed.

**2 What is the likely cause of the injury?** Fractures of the proximal tibia are unusual, especially in adult animals. Trauma is the most likely cause, possibly a fall or an awkward landing after jumping. The bone density appears adequate on this view, but a lateral view and radiographs of the contralateral limb should be taken to rule out the possibility of a pathological aetiology.

**3 How could this problem be treated and managed?** Successful reduction of this type of fracture is difficult and cannot be achieved closed. Internal fixation can be attempted but does require orthopaedic surgical skills. Amputation of the limb is an alternative depending on the circumstances and the client's wishes.

If surgery is attempted, an approach can be made craniomedially over the stifle joint, displacing the patella medially (168b). Reconstruction of the articular surface by placing a 1.5 mm lag screw is the first consideration. A 3 mm intramedullary pin can then be placed normograde from the base of the tibial crest through the

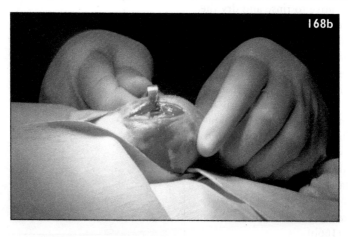

168b

medullary cavity of the proximal fragments to that of the distal tibia. Some of the smaller fragments are irreducible; therefore, the limb will need considerable support (heavy full limb bandage that does not hyperextend the stifle) for several weeks following surgery. Good pre- and postoperative analgesia is essential. In the immediate perioperative period, both opioids (e.g. morphine, methadone or buprenorphine) and NSAIDs (e.g. meloxicam or carprofen) are indicated. Continued NSAID therapy should be given for at least 7–14 days, or longer if necessary. Exercise should be severely restricted (by cage resting) for 4–6 weeks and then slowly returned to normal over the following 6 weeks. Follow-up radiographs 6–8 weeks after the surgery are recommended to assess healing.

**4 What long-term considerations should be discussed with the owner following surgical treatment?** Implant removal may need to be considered in the longer term, although in most cases the pins and screws are left in place. Unless the articular surface is perfectly congruous, which is difficult to achieve, there is an increased risk of degenerative joint changes occurring in the left stifle following this type of injury.

## CASE 169

**1 What viral infections are rabbits routinely vaccinated against in the UK?** Myxomatosis virus and viral haemorrhagic disease (VHD) virus.

**2 Describe how the vaccination is administered and onset of immunity.** The vaccine is a recombinant attenuated myxoma vector virus which contains the RHD VP60 capsid gene such that a single vaccine immunises against the two diseases (**169**). The vaccine is administered subcutaneously and provides immunity for 1 year. Full onset of immunity takes 3 weeks to develop.

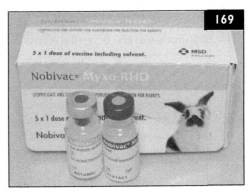

**3 At what age can rabbits be vaccinated?** Rabbits can be vaccinated from 5 weeks of age.

**4 Are there any situations in which their use is contraindicated?** Vaccination is not recommended in the first 14 days of pregnancy. There is also no safety study performed on breeding bucks to prove or disprove effects on fertility.

## CASE 170

This rabbit has a palpably enlarged liver (170). Which biochemical parameters may be used in the rabbit in the assessment of liver disease?

- *GGT* – is found in the liver and kidney, but GGT of renal origin is not found in the circulation. Therefore, serum GGT is all of hepatic origin, and levels will be raised with hepatocellular damage and biliary stasis.
- *AST* – is found in the liver, cardiac and skeletal muscle, kidney and pancreas, with highest levels in the liver and skeletal muscle. Elevation of AST will be seen with conditions causing hepatocellular necrosis.
- *ALP* – activity originates from many tissues, including bone, intestine, kidney and placenta as well as liver, with highest levels in intestine and kidney. The highest levels of ALP activity in the liver are found in the membranes bordering the bile canaliculi, and levels increase in conditions of biliary stasis. Rabbits have two liver ALP isoenzymes.
- *ALT* – is of limited use for evaluating hepatic damage in the rabbit, as it has little tissue specificity. For example, ALT activity in rabbit heart muscle and liver is similar, and rabbit liver has only half the ALT activity of that in the dog. The half-life of ALT is only 5 hours in the rabbit, compared with 45–60 hours in the dog. However, significant elevations in ALT can be found in conditions of hepatic damage and necrosis such as hepatic coccidiosis and hepatic lipidosis.
- *Bilirubin and bile acids* – the main product of haem breakdown in the rabbit is biliverdin, although some is converted to bilirubin, which is present at measurable levels. Biliverdin assays are not commercially available. Serum bilirubin levels reflect hepatocellular and biliary tree function. Visible icterus is a rare presenting sign in the rabbit. Significant hyperbilirubinaemia is usually associated with biliary obstruction and cholestasis (e.g. neoplasia of the biliary tree and hepatic coccidiosis). Bile acids (cholic acid and chenodeoxycholic acid) are synthesized in the liver from cholesterol, and they are essential for fat digestion and absorption. There is normally a highly efficient enterohepatic circulation of bile acids, and blood levels will rise only if liver function is impaired. There is little information on the use of bile acids as an indicator of liver function in the rabbit, but it is presumed that it will be a sensitive indicator, as in other species. As the rabbit is a herbivore and always has ingesta in its GI tract, the taking of fasting and postprandial levels is not practical.
- *Total serum protein levels* vary in rabbits with breed and age. The albumin fraction is approximately 60%, higher than for most other mammals. Hypoproteinaemia will occur in rabbits with significant liver disease, due to decreased production.

## CASE 171
**What potential toxin might these contain, and what clinical signs might it cause in the rabbit?** Mycotoxins (e.g. aflatoxin produced by *Aspergillus flavus*) can be found in mouldy feeds. These are toxic metabolites of fungi. These toxins can cause gastroenteritis and liver toxicity in rabbits, leading to clinical signs including diarrhoea, anorexia and collapse. Subclinical intoxication may affect the immune system, resulting in immunosuppression. This in turn may predispose the rabbit to developing bacterial infections.

## CASE 172
**What advice would you give an owner wishing to use preventive flea products on a pet rabbit?** Preventive flea treatment is rarely indicated in domestic rabbits. Treatment is usually required in response to fleas being seen on the rabbit. *Spillopsyllus cuniculi*, the rabbit flea, is an important vector for myxomatosis. Cat fleas can also occasionally live on rabbits. Products licensed for use in rabbits in the UK are imidacloprid and permethrin. Both kill adult fleas. The former lasts for 1 week and should be repeated every 4 weeks; the latter lasts for 2 weeks and treatment should be repeated fortnightly. The use of fipronil is contraindicated in rabbits following adverse reactions to both the spray and the spot-on preparations in small and young animals. Fatalities have occurred. Other side effects seen include depression and anorexia.

## CASE 173
**1 Describe the abnormality.** There is kyphosis of the spine at the thoracolumbar junction and the vertebral body of T12 is abnormal in shape (small and wedge-shaped). A ventrodorsal radiograph also revealed an abnormally shaped L1 vertebral body; it appeared wider than normal and asymmetrical.
**2 What is the most likely cause of this problem?** Differential diagnoses for bilateral hindlimb paresis include spinal fracture (often at the level of L7), intervertebral disc disease, congenital anomalies, spinal abscesses and spinal neoplasia. Given the age of the patient, the radiographic appearance of the spine and the chronicity of the clinical signs, this is most likely a congenital disorder.
**3 What other diagnostic test could be performed to confirm the diagnosis?** Myelography should be performed to assess whether the abnormality detected on radiography is causing significant compression of the spinal cord. In some rabbits, kyphosis or scoliosis is an incidental finding and the radiograph alone does not confirm that this spinal abnormality is the cause of the observed clinical signs.

Magnetic resonance imaging (MRI) can also be used to assess the spinal cord.

**4 Discuss treatment options.** The treatment options for congenital spinal disease are limited. Depending on the results of myelography/MRI, spinal surgery may be a challenging consideration. Analgesia can be a useful medical adjunct. Options include opioids, opioid-like drugs (e.g. tramadol) and NSAIDS (e.g. meloxicam). The latter provide anti-inflammatory benefits in addition to analgesia.

**5 What is the prognosis?** The prognosis in this case is likely to be poor, especially if treatment does not ameliorate the clinical signs. Prolonged hindlimb paresis can interfere with caecotrophy and grooming and therefore lead to dermatopathies and GI disease. If urinary incontinence develops, secondary perineal urine scalding may occur. The paresis usually progresses to paralysis with time, as it did 6 months after initial presentation in this rabbit, at which point euthanasia is recommended.

## CASE 174

**Which antibiotic drugs are known to be safe to use in rabbits, and by what route should they be administered?** A wide range of antibiotics are available (**174**). Potentiated sulfonamides are relatively non-toxic in rabbits and diffuse well into body tissues. They are easy to administer, being available as both injectable and oral preparations. They have not been reported as causing enteritis in rabbits. They have a wide range of activity including activity against *Toxoplasma* spp. and *Coccidia* spp. Dose rates in rabbits range from 15–30 mg/kg p/o or s/c q12h. Tissue necrosis may occur with subcutaneous injection of this drug, and for this reason the authors prefer oral administration.

Fluoroquinolones have activity against Gram-negative and some Gram-positive organisms. In the UK enrofloxacin is licensed for use in rabbits and comes in both an injectable and an oral form. It is active against *Pasteurella multocida*, *Pseudomonas* spp. and some *Mycoplasma* spp., but it is not active against anaerobes and is therefore not the drug of choice in the treatment of rabbit abscesses. The dose rate in rabbits is 5 mg/kg p/o q12h. Caution should be used when prescribing this

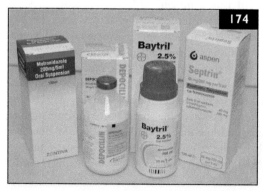

drug in pregnant or lactating rabbits, as there is an absence of data on its use in these circumstances. Enrofloxacin is particularly useful in the treatment of respiratory and GI tract infections. When given by s/c or i/m injection, it may cause a localized tissue reaction, muscle necrosis and sterile abscess formation. There is evidence that it may cause arthropathies in juvenile rabbits. It does not cause enteritis in rabbits. Overuse of this drug in rabbits is a major issue and bacterial resistances have been reported.

Tetracyclines are bacteriostatic antibiotics and have a relatively broad spectrum of activity, including activity against *Mycoplasma* spp., *Chlamydophila* spp., some protozoa and many Gram-positive and Gram-negative bacteria. However, many organisms are resistant to tetracyclines, including *Staphylococcus aureus*. They may be given both orally and parenterally; however, they are unpalatable and may not reach therapeutic levels if given in the drinking water. At high doses (30 mg/kg q8h) the injectable form may induce diarrhoea. Tetracycline is poorly absorbed from the GI tract and is therefore useful in the treatment of GI bacterial infections. Dose rates of 50 mg/kg p/o q8–12h have been described.

Metronidazole is a bactericidal antibiotic with activity against anaerobic Gram-positive bacteria and most Gram-negative bacteria. It is relatively non-toxic and may be administered both orally and parenterally. It is indicated in the treatment of *Clostridium spiroforme* enterotoxaemia. A dose rate of 40 mg/kg p/o q24h for 3 days has been reported.

Penicillin and cephalosporin antibiotics may be used in rabbits, but only if given parenterally. Animals should be carefully monitored for evidence of GI disturbance (e.g. diarrhoea) and the owner warned of these potential side effects. Treatment should be stopped if this occurs. Concurrent administration of probiotics may be of some benefit. Penicillin and cephalosporin have good activity against anaerobes and are therefore useful in the treatment of rabbit abscesses. They should not be given orally, since they may induce antibiotic-associated enterotoxaemia and death.

## CASE 175

**1 What species of tick most commonly infects domestic rabbits?** *Haemaphysalis leporispalustris* (the continental rabbit tick).
**2 For what diseases can ticks act as vectors?** Myxomatosis, papillomatosis, tularaemia (not UK).
**3 How would you treat tick infection in a rabbit?** Manual removal is the preferred treatment. Pyrethroid-containing topical products may also be used, for example, Xenex Ultra spot on (Genetrix) which is licensed in the UK for use in rabbits.

## CASE 176

**What secondary problems are associated with obesity in pet rabbits (176)?** Pet rabbits are commonly found to be obese if they are fed an inappropriate diet or *ad libitum* pellets or they get inadequate exercise. Obesity can predispose to hypertension, cardiac hypertrophy, hepatic lipidosis, exacerbation of arthritic conditions, cystitis, hypercalciuria and urine scald involving the perineum.

Obese rabbits are also less able to groom themselves properly. This may result in accumulation of matted caecotrophs around the perineum, which predisposes to fly strike (myiasis). In addition, obesity increases the risk of anaesthetic complications and therefore adversely affects the prognosis for rabbits requiring surgery. If an appropriate diet is fed (unlimited access to fresh meadow hay, grass, green leafy vegetables and some fruit and root vegetables), obesity is rare.

## CASE 177
**What is this object?** A starch grain.
The likely source is from a powdered latex examination glove.

## CASE 178
**1 How would you differentiate peripheral versus central disease in this rabbit?** A thorough neurological examination may elucidate whether the head tilt is due to a central or peripheral lesion; however, further diagnostics, such as skull radiographs or a CT scan, may be required for definitive localization.
**2 List your differentials for a head tilt in a rabbit.** Differential diagnoses for a head tilt include peripheral disease, such as otitis interna affecting the vestibulocochlear nerve (CN VIII), or central disease where the vestibular nuclei within the brainstem may be affected. A head tilt, circling and rolling may all be present with both central and peripheral disease. Conscious proprioception and postural reactions, on the other hand, will typically be abnormal (either weak or absent) with brainstem disease. They should be normal and present with peripheral disease. Other differentials include trauma, *Encephalitozoon cuniculi*, cerebral larval migrans of *Baylisascaris procyonis*, a severe tooth root abscess that has affected the inner ear or brain, toxins and thromboembolic disease.
**3 Given the history with this rabbit, what is the most likely cause of disease?** In the young rabbit with potential exposure to raccoon faeces in its feed, the most likely differential is *B. procyonis*. *Baylisascaris* eggs are highly resistant in the environment and can remain infective for over a year. The egg is ingested. The larva is released into the intestine and then burrows through the intestinal mucosa and migrates throughout the body, with a predilection for the central nervous system, where it causes encephalomalacia. Larvae may also migrate through and cause substantial damage to the liver and eyes. Unfortunately, there is no method for antemortem diagnosis of *Baylisascaris* larval migrans, and thus successful treatment methods have not been determined.

## CASE 179

**1 How would you diagnose haematuria in the rabbit?** Rabbit urine can contain porphyrin pigments. These colour the urine dark brown to red and this colouration is often confused by owners with blood. Haematuria may be diagnosed either by using a urine dipstick, with a positive reaction, or by examination of the urine sediment for red blood cells. Examination of the urine under a Wood's lamp can distinguish between the two conditions, although this is rarely necessary in clinical practice. Porphyrin pigments will fluoresce, whereas haemoglobin does not.

**2 What are the differential diagnoses for this condition?** Differential diagnoses for haematuria include reproductive tract disease (uterine adenocarcinoma, uterine polyps, abortion and endometrial venous aneurysm) and urinary tract disease (cystitis, bladder polyps, pyelonephritis, renal infarcts, urolithiasis).

**3 What further tests would you perform to reach a diagnosis?** A thorough history should be sought and a full clinical examination undertaken prior to obtaining a sterile urine sample, either by catheterization under sedation or by cystocentesis, for analysis and culture. Radiography and ultrasonography may be used to investigate whether lesions are associated with the genital or reproductive tract. Contrast studies may be indicated with urinary tract disease. Laboratory tests such as full haematology and biochemistry should be carried out.

## CASE 180

**1 What is the most likely cause of the alopecia?** The most likely cause of the alopecia is exfoliative dermatitis as a paraneoplastic syndrome associated with thymoma or thymic lymphoma.

**2 How would you confirm your diagnosis?** A dermatological work-up consisting of microscopic examination of skin scrapes, hair plucks and tape strips would rule out ectoparasites. The presence of a thoracic mass could be confirmed using ultrasonographic, radiographic or computed tomography imaging techniques.

**3 What treatment options are available?** Treatment options include euthanasia, thoracotomy to remove the mediastinal mass (in feline species dermatological signs have been shown to resolve following mass removal) or localized radiation therapy.

## CASE 181

**1 What determines the maximum fixator pin diameter that should be used?** The diameter of the fixator pins should not exceed 20% of the diameter of the fractured bone. Negative-profile Ellis pins provide a thread without increasing the diameter of the pin.

2 For smaller patients, what alternative materials can be used to construct external fixation that is equally rigid and resistant to chewing? Kirschner wires or hypodermic needles may be used as external fixator pins in small rabbits or in the treatment of fractures of very small bones. The material should be smooth, and three or four pins per segment are usually required for adequate fixation. The connecting bar is positioned approximately 1 cm (0.4 inch) away from the skin (allowing for some postoperative swelling) and it can be fashioned from bone cement or acrylics in cases where standard clamps and bars are considered too large and bulky.

3 What factors affect the optimal time of removal of an external fixator in these patients? The three major factors that influence the timing of pin removal are the type of fracture, the age of the animal and the degree of vascular disruption of the tissues. It is often advantageous to stage the removal of the apparatus if possible, as this increases load bearing while the fracture heals. As a general rule, fixator removal at 6–8 weeks post surgery is suitable for most fracture types and patients.

## CASE 182

1 What is the causative agent, and how is it transmitted? The causative agent for rabbit syphilis is *Treponema cuniculi*, a spirochaete. It is spread by the venereal route and by direct contact. Affected does can infect kits as they pass through the birth canal. There can be a symptomless carrier state, and overt disease is precipitated by stress.

2 How is the condition diagnosed? Clinical signs of vesicles, ulcers, scabs and proliferative lesions around the genitals and face (from autoinoculation) are highly suggestive. Definitive diagnosis involves identification of the organism. A deep scrape of the lesions can reveal the organism when viewed microscopically using a dark field background. Skin biopsies stained with silver stains may also be used.

3 What treatment can be used? The treatment of choice is with systemic penicillin. Penicillin G benzathine (42,000–84,000 IU/kg s/c q7d for 3 weeks) is the most commonly used regime.

4 What precautions should be taken when administering this drug to a rabbit? The rabbit should be monitored closely for signs of antibiotic-associated enterotoxaemia, such as diarrhoea. Signed consent should be obtained from the owner for use of this drug, as it is not licensed in rabbits. The drug should always be given parenterally and not orally. Once-weekly dosing also reduces the risk of toxicity developing. The use of probiotics while the animal is undergoing treatment may be beneficial. It is essential that the rabbit is fed a healthy diet consisting of grass, fresh hay and leafy vegetables.

## CASE 183

**What are your differential diagnoses?** Differential diagnoses for urinary incontinence include: lumbosacral vertebral fractures; vertebral disease (e.g. intervertebral disc prolapse, spondylosis), CNS disease secondary to infection with *Encephalitozoon cuniculi*, hormone responsive urinary incontinence in ovariohysterectomized female rabbits, urinary calculi, hypercalciuria and urinary tract infection. Any condition that may result in weakness of the hindlimbs could in theory present as urinary scalding, because the rabbit would be unable to posture correctly when urinating. Weakness of the hindlimbs may occur with systemic disease such as septicaemia, liver failure, renal failure, hepatic lipidosis and cardiovascular disease.

## CASE 184

**Why is this, and how are they thought to work in the rabbit?** Probiotics contain non-pathogenic microorganisms. These compete with pathogenic bacteria for nutrients and space, so inhibiting pathogenic bacterial growth. Probiotic products usually contain yeasts, *Lactobacillus* spp. and *Enterococcus* spp. In rabbits, however, the predominant species of caecal bacteria are *Bacteroides* spp. and *Lactobacillus* spp. is generally absent. This raises the question as to whether supplementing with predominately *Lactobacillus* compounds is beneficial to rabbits. Microorganisms are easily killed by the acid in the stomach, so microencapsulated products should be used. Probiotics are unlikely to be harmful; they are only beneficial or ineffective. Therefore, they may be useful in the treatment of GI disease in rabbits.

## CASE 185

**1 What is your diagnosis?** Dystocia. Cases of dystocia are extremely rare in rabbits. They are predisposed by fetal oversize, obesity, small pelvic anatomy and uterine inertia.

**2 What are the likely clinical signs associated with this condition?** Clinical signs of dystocia include non-productive straining, steady contractions and a bloody or greenish-black discharge from the vagina.

**3 What treatment options are available?** If these clinical signs are present and vaginal delivery is not possible, then a caesarian section is the treatment of choice. In this case, lubrication and gentle traction resulted in a successful delivery of the kit.

## CASE 186

**1 What abnormality can you detect?** The stomach is considerably distended with the caudal border extending well beyond the reach of the last rib, in to the mid-abdominal region. There is gas present within the stomach.

**2 What is the likely cause of this problem?** This is due to decreased gastric motility (gastric stasis) causing dehydration and impaction of the normal stomach contents (food, caecotrophs and ingested hair from grooming). This could be complicated by a partial or full obstruction of the pylorus or proximal duodenum, affecting the outflow of the stomach.

Motility can be decreased for many reasons, including a low-fibre diet, dehydration, anorexia, stress and pain. In long-haired breeds such as Angoras, excessive ingestion of hair can be the cause of a hairball. With this case, the Dwarf Lop rabbit was moulting and hair ingestion was thought to play a role in development of the condition.

**3 How would you treat it?** Treatment is aimed at rehydration, analgesia and supportive care. Rabbits should be hospitalized in quiet surroundings away from potential predators to minimize stress. Treatment consists of the following:

- *Fluid therapy* – to maintain circulation and rehydrate GI contents. In mild cases, oral fluids may be all that is required, but in more severe cases intravenous fluids are indicated. Maintenance volumes are 100 ml/kg/day.
- *Analgesia* – buprenorphine (0.01–0.05 mg/kg s/c or i/v q8h), butorphanol (0.1–0.5 mg/kg s/c or i/v q2–4h), carprofen (2–4 mg/kg s/c or i/v q24h).
- *Motility modifiers* (contraindicated if a blockage is suspected) – metoclopramide (0.5 mg/kg s/c q12h); cisapride (0.5 mg/kg p/o q12h); ranitidine (2–5 mg/kg p/o q12–24h).
- *Assisted feeding* – commercially available high-fibre herbivore recovery diets, slurries of ground rabbit pellets, vegetable baby foods. Always offer hay.
- *Exercise* – helps to stimulate GI motility.
- *Antibiotics* – are not indicated in the treatment of gut stasis.
- *Surgical intervention* – may be required with a gastrotomy to empty the stomach contents in cases of gastric distension unresponsive to medical treatment. With this case, the rabbit responded to medical treatment over a 3-day period, going on to make a full recovery.

## CASE 187

**1 What are the key parameters that should be monitored?** As a general principle, as much information as possible should be gathered for as long as the rabbit requires or tolerates it. Therefore, if the rabbit is still intubated (**187a**), it is possible to acquire expired carbon dioxide readings (using capnography) as well as oxygen saturation (pulse oximeter) and possibly non-invasive blood pressure measurements

(Doppler, sphygmomanometer and cuff). However, for most rabbits extubation should be swift on administration of any anaesthetic reversal agent, or turning off of anaesthetic vapours, and this will limit the parameters that can be monitored.

Extubated rabbits recovering from an anaesthetic should be monitored for respiratory rate, heart rate, temperature and reflexes (**187b, c**).

**2 With what frequency should parameters be recorded?** Parameters should be initially recorded every 5 minutes as an extension of the anaesthetic monitoring regime. When the rabbit shows response to further stimuli such as the pedal reflex or even lifting its head, then parameters could be recorded at 15- to 30-minute intervals.

**3 When would it be deemed appropriate to remove a recovering rabbit from an incubator or away from heat support, and when should postoperative monitoring cease?** The main aim is to ensure that the rabbit is able to maintain its body position in dorsal recumbency and that its body temperature is stabilized or returned to baseline (pre-anaesthetic) normal values (38.5–40.0 °C). However, sudden changes in environmental temperature and/or removing the rabbit from a controlled temperature environment, such as that provided by an incubator, too soon can result in prolonged recoveries due to

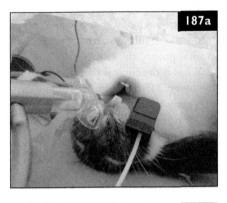

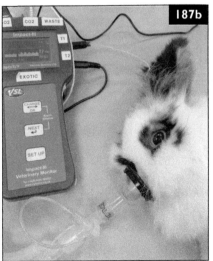

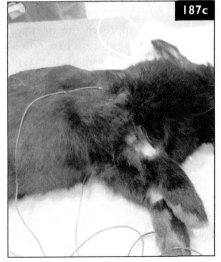

low body temperatures. It is advisable to return the environmental temperature to normal room temperature (21 °C) gradually and assess the rabbit's thermoregulatory ability by checking the rectal temperature 10–15 minutes after a change has occurred. When the rabbit has demonstrated the ability to maintain a stable body temperature that matches baseline values, it can be returned to its hospital cage and then another rectal temperature check can be assessed a further 10–15 minutes later. Following this check and evidence of purposeful movement, the postoperative monitoring can stop. It must always remain an option and you should always be prepared to return the rabbit to the incubator, or similar, if its body temperature falls.

## CASE 188

**1 Describe what you see in the ultrasound scan (188).** There is a large solitary, thin-walled subcapsular cortical cystic lesion, filled with anechoic fluid at the cranial pole of the kidney.

**2 What is the clinical significance of this lesion, and what advice would you give to the owner?** Renal cysts in rabbits are not usually associated with clinical signs and may only be detected at postmortem examination. They are inherited in rabbits as an autosomal recessive trait and the owner should be advised not to breed from this animal.

As a precaution, urinalysis and serum biochemistry can be performed to assess kidney health.

## CASE 189

**How do you approach the treatment of dental abscesses?** Many methods of dealing with these abscesses are proposed, and many practitioners have developed their own favoured method. To maximize the chance of a successful outcome, the following procedures should be undertaken:

- Carry out radiography or computed tomography of the skull to assess the extent of tooth and bone involvement.
- Surgically remove the abscess and abscess capsule, in its entirety if possible.
- Remove all dental fragments associated with the abscess.
- Debride all infected/necrotic bone.
- Obtain a bacterial culture and sensitivity to identify the causative organism(s).
- Administer both local and systemic antibiosis, based on bacterial sensitivity results.

Unfortunately, in many situations one or several of these criteria cannot be met. The administration of local treatment can be achieved in several ways:

- *AIPPMA beads.* The placement of antibiotic-impregnated polymethylmethacrylate (AIPMMA) beads allows high antibiotic levels locally with very little systemic absorption. Appropriate systemic antibiotics are also given for at least 2 weeks postoperatively. Bone cement may be purchased and an appropriate antibiotic added (e.g. 1 g gentamicin powder is added to 20 g PMMA). Bone cement with antibiotic already incorporated may also be purchased, which can then be made into appropriate size beads. Premade beads are available but these are generally too large for rabbits.
- *Doxycycline gel* provides a slow release formulation of local doxycycline. It is formulated for the treatment of periodontal disease.
- *Sodium hydroxyapatite.* This is synthetic bone powder and can be used to fill large bony deficits, where it acts as a scaffold for bone regrowth. Technically, it is contraindicated in infected sites but anecdotal reports from practitioners in the USA and UK have reported very good success by mixing it with an antibiotic powder (e.g. penicillin).

Opinions vary on whether it is best to close the surgical site after the local antibiosis is instilled, or to leave it open so that further treatment can be administered. Rabbit pus does not drain, so leaving the wound open is not for drainage purposes. In general, when using AIPPMA beads or sodium hydroxyapatite, it is necessary for practical reasons to close the wound to prevent loss of the implant. Some practitioners prefer not to use implants; instead they marsupialize the surgical site to allow continued flushing of the wound and repeated instillations of local antibiosis. The wound is allowed to heal by secondary intention. This does allow more control over continued treatment of the affected area and easier monitoring and detection of recurrence.

Postoperative analgesia should always be given. Systemic antibiotics may need to be given for several weeks or months.

## CASE 190

**1 What can cause renal failure in rabbits?** Renal failure in rabbits may occur secondary to pyelonephritis and infection with *Pasteurella multocida* or *Staphylococcus* spp. *Encephalitozoon cuniculi* is a common cause of chronic interstitial nephritis. Non-infectious causes include hypercalcaemia; renal calcinosis secondary to hypervitaminosis D and hypercalcaemia; neoplasia and nephrotoxins.

**2 How would you treat this condition?** Treatment for renal failure includes supportive care and parenteral fluid therapy to promote increased urine output. Intravenous lactated Ringer's solution is ideal. If dehydrated, replace the deficit over 6 hours and then switch to maintenance fluids of 100 ml/kg/day once BUN concentrations reach normal values. Once dehydration is corrected and the rabbit is urinating normally, s/c fluids may be used instead of i/v fluids. Serum potassium levels should be carefully monitored. General supportive care with syringe feeding, B-complex vitamins, probiotics and intestinal stimulant drugs may be indicated. Anabolic steroid or human recombinant erythropoietin therapy may be beneficial. ACE inhibitors such as benazepril, which is licensed for use in cases of chronic renal insufficiency in cats in the UK, may also be beneficial in rabbits. Dose rates of 0.1–0.5 mg/kg p/o q24h have prolonged survival times in rabbits diagnosed with renal disease. Antibiotics may be indicated in cases associated with pyelonephritis or infectious disease. Tetracyclines, aminoglycosides and trimethoprim/sulfonamide combinations should be avoided, as these are potentially nephrotoxic. However, as in most species, the prognosis is guarded.

## CASE 191

**1 To what secondary parasitic condition is this rabbit susceptible (191a)?** Fly strike (myiasis) (**191b**).

**2 How would you treat an affected rabbit?** Urgent treatment is necessary for rabbits suffering from myiasis, as affected rabbits can rapidly succumb to toxic shock. Supportive care (fluid therapy, analgesics and assisted feeding) and antibiotics should be given. The rabbit should have all the caked faecal/caecotroph material and surrounding fur clipped away. Maggots must be manually removed or flushed out with dilute antiseptic solution. Systemic ivermectin may be given (0.4 mg/kg s/c) to kill any internal or deep subcutaneous maggots that cannot be removed, or any that subsequently hatch from unremoved eggs. Topical antiseptic creams (e.g. silver sulfadiazine) may be applied. There may be large skin deficits and deep wounds that require attention for several days or weeks. It is essential to determine and

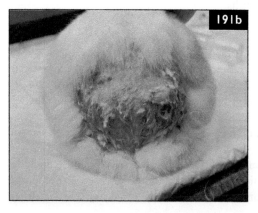

address the underlying cause of the accumulated caecotrophs/diarrhoea/urine scalding that initially attracted the flies.

**3 What husbandry advice would you give the owner?** Prevention of further episodes is by frequent examination of the ventrum of the rabbit, fly control and regular clipping/cleaning of the perineal region if necessary. In predisposed animals there are licensed veterinary products in the

UK that can be applied topically to act as a deterrent for flies (e.g. Xenex Ultra Spot-On [active ingredient permethrin] and Rearguard [active ingredient cypromazine]).

The hutch should be cleaned out regularly to ensure a clean, dry bed and, if possible, litter training of the rabbit should be performed. Reducing the risk of obesity with regular exercise and an ideal diet will also reduce the amount of time the rabbit spends sitting in one place. Fly screens and strips can be used around the enclosure, or the rabbit could be brought indoors to reduce the risk of exposure to flies.

## CASE 192

**1 What are the possible causes?** There are many possible causes of abortion in does. These include infection (bacterial, fungal, viral, parasitic), trauma, stress, toxins, genetic causes and dietary deficiencies (e.g. vitamin E, vitamin A, protein). *Listeria monocytogenes* has been known to cause late abortion in rabbits and should be considered in this case.

**2 How would you investigate this case?** It is vital to obtain a thorough clinical history from the owner. Information on previous litters, other cases of abortion, recent changes to the environment and recent drug treatment should be gathered. The doe should have a thorough clinical examination and be checked for any retained fetuses. Fetus and placenta should be submitted for histopathological examination and culture.

## CASE 193

**1 How can non-obstructive and obstructive ileus be differentiated from each other?** The table summarizes the differences between non-obstructive and obstructive ileus.

| Observations | Non-obstructive ileus | Obstructive ileus |
|---|---|---|
| Clinical signs | Gradual onset (days to weeks) | Sudden onset (24–48 hours) |
| | Gradual reduction in faecal size and output | Faecal output stops suddenly |
| | Crave fibre | Severe depression |
| | Initially bright, gradual onset of depression and abdominal pain | Abdominal pain |
| | | Reluctance to move |
| | | Shock – slow capillary refill time, pale mucous membranes |
| | Mild to moderate dehydration | Severe dehydration |
| | | Death in 24–48 hours |

*Continued*

| Observations | Non-obstructive ileus | Obstructive ileus |
|---|---|---|
| Radiographic findings | Compacted material in stomach and sometimes caecum, often with halo of gas<br>As symptoms progress, entire GI tract gas-filled. Stomach usually last to bloat<br>Fluid only present late in disease | Fluid and gas present cranial to obstruction<br>Bubbles of gas in stomach, no halo<br>If caecal obstruction, fluid and bubbles of air in caecum |

**2 How does their treatment differ?** Treatment of non-obstructive ileus is medical and aimed at supporting the rabbit and restoring normal motility. Treatment consists of fluid therapy, analgesia, motility modifiers, assisted feeding and gentle exercise.

Obstructive ileus is a surgical emergency. Rabbits will develop true obstructions with dried ingesta, hair ('trichobezoars') and ingested foreign materials such as carpet, rubber or plastic. The most common sites are the pylorus, proximal duodenum and ileocaecocolic region. Occasionally, just the caecum can be obstructed. Rarely, neoplasia, abscesses or surgical adhesions can cause obstruction. The rabbit should first be stabilized with fluid therapy, warmth and analgesia. Metoclopramide, cisapride and ranitidine are contraindicated prior to surgery, but are useful postoperatively to stimulate GI motility. Postoperative analgesia, fluid therapy and nutritional support are vital to maximize the chance of success.

## CASE 194

**1 What condition is seen in this rabbit (194)?** Plantar pododermatitis ('hock burn'), a chronic, ulcerative, granulomatous dermatitis of the plantar surface of the metatarsals. It is sometimes also seen on the volar surface of the metacarpals. Dermatitis of the plantar skin becomes ulcerated and secondarily infected with *Staphylococcus aureus* or other bacteria. The infection can progress into the underlying tissue and may result in osteomyelitis and septicaemia.

**2 List the predisposing factors to the development of this condition.** Predisposing factors of podermatitis include obesity; inactivity; dirty wet bedding; grid flooring/ rough flooring; frequent thumping and bruising of the foot and breed (Rex breeds predisposed as no guard hairs).

**3 How would you treat it?** The lesions should be debrided and cleaned with antiseptic solution. Systemic antibiosis (preferably based on culture and sensitivity) should be instigated. Topical treatment of Sudocrem can be applied to the area to act as a protective barrier and to reduce inflammation.

NSAIDs such as meloxicam should be given. If the lesions are deep, radiography should be undertaken to assess if osteomyelitis is present. Dressings may be applied to protect the area; they are well tolerated by some rabbits but rapidly chewed off by others. In the latter case an Elizabethan collar may be appropriate, but this may be poorly tolerated and will prevent caecotrophy. The rabbit should be housed on soft, dry bedding such as synthetic sheepskin, 'vet-bed' or deep hay, and predisposing husbandry issues must be addressed. Resolution may be difficult to achieve and the prognosis is guarded if osteomyelitis is present.

## CASE 195

**1 What is the likely diagnosis?** Pregnancy toxaemia occurs in the last week of gestation in rabbits and is predisposed by obesity, stress, environmental changes, poor quality diets and periods of anorexia.

**2 What is the prognosis?** The prognosis in this case is poor and treatment can be unrewarding. The rabbit should be kept warm and given i/v fluids and calcium gluconate. Critical care food should be syringe fed once the patient is able to eat and swallow. Intensive supportive care should be given with intestinal stimulant drugs and oral fluids. The condition can be prevented by avoiding the predisposing factors in late pregnancy.

The use of corticosteroids to treat shock is controversial and is down to clinician preference. Steroids should always be used with care in rabbits because they can induce fatal hepatopathies.

## CASE 196

**1 What are the differential diagnoses?** Differential diagnoses include cystic mastitis, mammary dysplasia, mammary adenocarcinoma, pseudopregnancy, normal lactation and septic mastitis. Cystic mammary glands are often associated with uterine hyperplasia and uterine adenocarcinoma in older intact does. They may also progress and eventually become malignant mammary adenocarcinomas. These spread locally and may metastasize to the regional lymph nodes, lungs and other organs.

**2 What further diagnostic tests are indicated?** Further diagnostic tests should include fine-needle aspirate of the mass for cytological examination, punch or excisional biopsy, radiography and ultrasonography of the reproductive tract in entire does. Thoracic radiographs should also be taken in cases of mammary adenocarcinoma.

**3 What treatment is indicated?** The treatment of choice for non-infectious cystic mastitis is ovariohysterectomy, with clinical signs resolving 3–4 weeks post surgery. Surgical excision of mammary tumours is indicated. There is evidence that early neutering of female rabbits decreases the risk of mammary tumour formation later in life. In this case the mass was removed and sent for histological examination at the same time as the ovariohysterectomy was performed.

## CASE 197

Name two poxvirus skin diseases of rabbits. For each one, describe the natural host and the clinical signs in both the natural host and the domestic rabbit.

1 *Myxomatosis.* Jungle rabbits (*Sylvilagus brasiliensis*) in Central and South America and Brush rabbits (*S. bachmani*) in California are the natural hosts in which the virus causes a cutaneous fibroma and no other systemic signs. In the domestic rabbit it

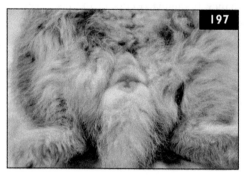

causes a fatal disease characterized by oedema of the head, ears, eyelids and genitalia (**197**), an oculonasal discharge and diffuse oedematous subcutaneous swellings (pseudotumours). Affected rabbits are pyrexic, lethargic and anorexic. Death is in about 14 days in an unvaccinated rabbit. Previously vaccinated rabbits may contract a milder form of the disease, with characteristic scabbing masses often on the bridge of the nose or around the eyes. It is believed that less virulent strains of the virus may also cause these milder signs, and these rabbits will usually survive.

2 *Shope fibroma virus.* The natural hosts are North and South American wild rabbits (*Sylvilagus* spp., e.g. *S. bachmani* and *S. floridanus*), in which no disease is produced. Domestic rabbits develop fibromas, which slough away after about 30 days. Newborn and young animals develop more extensive lesions than adults.

## CASE 198

1 **What are the differential diagnoses?** Differential diagnoses for testicular enlargement include orchitis and epididymitis secondary to bacterial infection, trauma, fight wounds, testicular neoplasia (seminoma, interstitial cell tumours, Sertoli cell tumours and teratomas) and testicular torsion.

2 **What is the treatment of choice?** Surgical castration is the treatment of choice, with histopathological examination of the affected tissue. If an infectious cause is

suspected, broad-spectrum systemic antibiotics should be commenced, based on results of culture and sensitivity. *Pasteurella multocida* infections are commonly found. *Treponema cuniculi* should also be considered.

## CASE 199

**What standard procedures should be considered prior to euthanasia in pet rabbits (199)?** Prior to euthanasia the owner should be told what to expect. How the procedure will be performed and arrangements for disposal of the body should be discussed. Arrangements should be made for the owner to be present if they request so. Veterinary personnel should be available to help restrain the animal, and reception staff should be notified that a rabbit is to be euthanased prior to arrival of the animal. A quiet room should be allocated for the procedure, preferably with a separate exit rather than through the waiting room.

Prior sedation of the animal is recommended, especially in fearful or aggressive rabbits, and this should be discussed with the owner. Placement of an i/v catheter into the rabbit's marginal ear vein will allow for smooth, trouble-free injection of the euthanasia agent. An extension T-port allows for easy administration of i/v drugs.

A topical local anaesthetic cream may be applied to the skin before catheter placement. The author's preference is to induce the rabbit, as if for anaesthetic, with propofol or alfaxalone i/v before injecting pentobarbitone by i/v. This prior anaesthetic agent significantly reduces the risk of any violent movements associated with reaction to the pentobarbitone prior to death. The owner should be warned that occasionally rabbits vocalize or gasp during euthanasia, although this is uncommon with the described approach.

A non-slip surface (such as a towel) should be provided on which to restrain the rabbit and the animal should be gently talked to and reassured during the procedure.

## CASE 200

**What surgical precautions should be taken to reduce the risk of these conditions developing in the postoperative period?** Handling of the abdominal organs should be minimal and done with great care, to avoid iatrogenic trauma and associated tearing of tissue and subsequent haemorrhage. Sterile saline should be used repeatedly to moisten the viscera and avoid desiccation of tissues that may predispose to adhesion formation. Surgical exposure time should be kept to a minimum. Copious abdominal lavage should be performed in all cases prior to closure of the abdomen to remove any blood clots or potential contamination from GI surgery. The calcium channel blocker verapamil (0.2 mg/kg p/o or i/v q8h for 9 doses) has been used in an experimental situation to reduce adhesion formation. Use of this drug might be indicated in cases where significant damage or irritation of the abdominal organs has occurred.

Gastrointestinal tract motility modifiers such as metoclopramide (0.5 mg/kg s/c or p/o q6–8h) and ranitidine (2–5 mg/kg p/o q12–24h) may be used perioperatively to reduce the risk of intestinal ileus. Suture materials should be carefully chosen and the size of suture material should be kept to a minimum. The use of catgut should be avoided in rabbits, as it is associated with a high risk of adhesion formation. Rabbits are more likely to react adversely to suture materials than other mammals, since their immune system reacts to form caseous material in response to foreign bodies and they are predisposed to adhesion formation. Monofilament synthetic suture material such as monofilament polyglyconate is preferred for use in rabbits, as it is made from polymers that are removed by hydrolytic breakdown rather than relying on phagocytosis and the rabbit's immune response to degrade. These are therefore less reactive and cause fewer and weaker adhesions.

## CASE 201
**What is the most likely cause of this lesion, and how would you treat it?** Acute cellulitis associated with bite wounds. *Pasteurella multocida* and *Staphylococcus aureus* are the commonest agents cultured, but other organisms may be involved (e.g. *Fusobacterium necrophorum*). The rabbit is likely to be febrile. Aggressive systemic therapy is required, preferably based on culture and sensitivity. NSAIDs such as meloxicam or carprofen should be given. Topical antiseptic or antibacterial creams may be applied (e.g. silver sulfadiazine). Supportive care is also important until the rabbit is eating and drinking normally (fluid therapy, assisted feeding, gut motility modifiers). The lesions may mature into an abscess, which will require surgical removal, or may heal to leave a large necrotic eschar, which will slough. Castration of both rabbits will reduce aggression, or the companion may need to be removed and the two live separately.

## CASE 202
**1 Describe the surgical techniques used to castrate male rabbits.** The rabbit is anaesthetized and placed in dorsal recumbency. After appropriate surgical preparation of the thin scrotal skin and surrounding area, an incision is made in one scrotum through the skin and parietal vaginal tunic (**202a**). Some surgeons prefer a single prescrotal incision rather that two separate scrotal incisions. The gubernaculum is manually torn to free the distal testis and epididymis (**202b**).

A ligature (using 3/0 absorbable suture material) is then placed around the testicular artery and vein, prior to removal of the testis and epididymis. As the inguinal ring remains open in rabbits, it is advisable to close the parietal vaginal tunic, usually with a single horizontal mattress suture. Alternatively, closed castration may be used. With this technique the parietal vaginal tunic is not incised, rather a transfixing ligature is placed around this and the spermatic cord, proximal to the testis, prior to excision of the testis (**202c**). The skin incision may be left open, with the edges apposed. If sutures are necessary in the skin, it is preferable to use an intradermal pattern (4/0 absorbable suture material). Tissue adhesives (e.g. cyanoacrylate glue) may be used, but excessive application may retard skin healing or stimulate self-trauma through grooming.

2 **What is the minimum recommended time post surgery that a male rabbit should be separated from its intact female companion?** The male may remain fertile for up to 6 weeks post castration and so should be physically separated from the intact doe until then. Indirect contact via a shared air space will aid a smooth reintroduction after this time.

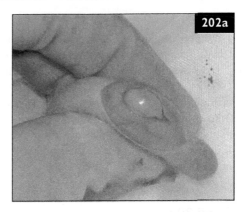

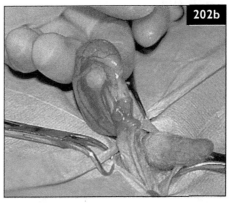

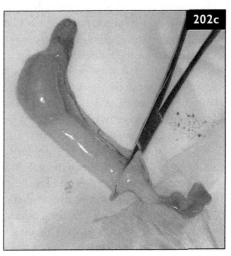

## CASE 203

**1 What ectoparasite is generally associated with these clinical signs (203)?**
*Cheyletiella parasitovorax* or, more rarely, *Leporacarus (Listrophorus) gibbus*.
**2 How would you treat this animal?** Ivermectin (0.2–0.4 mg/kg s/c every 10–14 days for 3 doses); topical selamectin (8–16 mg/kg once). Alternative treatments include topical permethrins and lime-sulfur dips.
**3 Are there any zoonotic implications?** Yes. *Cheyletiella parasitovorax* causes a papular dermatitis in man but cannot complete its life cycle on the human host. Effective treatment of the rabbit will resolve the problem. *Leporacarus gibbus* is not zoonotic.

## CASE 204

**What are the differential diagnoses for alopecia in the rabbit?** Differentials for alopecia in rabbits include cheyletiellosis; dermatophytosis; sarcoptic mange (rare – *S. scabiei* var. *cuniculi* and *N. cati* var. *cuniclui*); demodicosis; *Psorobia lagomorphae* infestation; sebaceous adenitis; barbering (by dominant or, more usually, subordinate companion); self-barbering (does in oestrus, associated with low-fibre diet); excessive grooming (compulsive behavioural problem); normal moult; pregnancy or pseudopregnancy (does pluck hair from dewlap and ventrum to line nest and expose nipples).

## CASE 205

**1 What is the treatment of choice, and what factors influence this decision?** While radiography is required for thorough assessment of the injury, based on the available information the treatment of choice is likely to be amputation of the affected limb. Open, contaminated fractures carry a very high risk of osteomyelitis and require aggressive surgical debridement if reduction and fixation are to be attempted. This is especially true if they present several days post trauma. Amputation reduces surgery time and the need for repeated check-ups, radiographs and bandage changes and therefore may be more suitable than other treatment options if the likelihood of adequate bone healing is poor, if the animal is particularly nervous and/or there are financial constraints.
**2 What is the prognosis?** The prognosis is good if amputation is carried out following prompt and adequate stabilization of the patient. Rabbits adapt very well to forelimb amputation and are able to ambulate soon after surgery. Once the fur grows back, the result is also aesthetically pleasing for an owner.
**3 Discuss pre- and postoperative considerations in such a case.** The patient must be stabilized prior to surgery. This may be achieved by the administration of i/v fluids, analgesia, prokinetics and antibiotics. Analgesia should be continued for

3–5 days postoperatively or until the rabbit is eating and defecating normally. Given the gross contamination of the wounds, a course of appropriate systemic antibiotics should be considered. Nutritional support is essential for all rabbits following major surgery and, after limb amputation, rabbits should be confined for a period of at least 7–10 days. During this time the wound should be monitored for seroma formation and signs of infection or dehiscence.

**4 What equipment would be required for the surgery?** A standard small mammal surgical kit and fine suture material are essential. If the amputation is to be performed by transecting the humerus (a common technique), it is advantageous to have a sharp hacksaw, an oscillating saw or a Gigli wire saw available. The use of crushing bone cutters is not appropriate, as rabbit bones have thin cortices and shatter readily. Bone wax is useful to plug the end of the bone. Alternative methods of amputation include removing the entire limb, including the scapula, which may produce a more cosmetic result, or dissection through the scapular–humeral joint.

## CASE 206

**What reflexes may be used in the assessment of anaesthetic depth in the rabbit?** The most useful reflexes in the rabbit are the pedal withdrawal reflex and the ear pinch response. The pedal withdrawal reflex involves extending the limb and pinching the web firmly to assess whether any limb withdrawal or muscle twitching is present. For surgical procedures, the hindlimb withdrawal should be absent or barely detectable. The forelimb withdrawal remains present at very deep planes of anaesthesia and it is not necessary for this reflex to be absent. The ear pinch response involves pinching the base of the ear (**206**). At light levels of anaesthesia the rabbit will shake its head. The palpebral reflex can be maintained at very deep levels of anaesthesia, so it is of limited use. It will be lost at lighter levels of anaesthesia if ketamine is used.

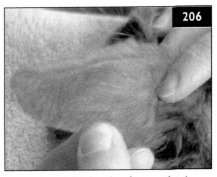

## CASE 207

**1 What radiographic changes are present and what is the most likely diagnosis given the signalment and clinical signs?** The radiographs show a nodular interstitial pattern of the lung field. The most likely diagnosis in a 7-year-old entire female rabbit is metastatic spread from a uterine adenocarcinoma. Abdominal radiography and ultrasonography revealed a large mass in the uterus.

**2 What differential diagnoses would you consider in a 7-year-old rabbit with these clinical signs?** Differential diagnoses for lower respiratory tract disease include: pneumonia; abscesses associated with pleuropneumonia; pleuropneumonia (secondary to infection with *Pasteurella multocida, Pseudomonas aeruginosa, Staphylococcus aureus, Bordetella bronchiseptica, Mycobacterium bovis, M. tuberculosis, Moraxella bovis, Francisella tularensis* and *Yersinia pestis*); primary thoracic neoplasia (thymoma); and secondary metastatic disease. Pleural effusion has been seen with cardiovascular disease (cardiomyopathy, valvular disease, pericarditis and atherosclerosis) and corona virus infection but this has not been reported as a spontaneous natural infection in pet rabbits.

**3 What is the prognosis?** The prognosis is grave and in this case the rabbit was euthanased.

**4 What preventive measures are there to reduce the incidence of this condition?** Ovariohysterectomy before the rabbit is 2 years old will reduce the incidence of this condition in female rabbits. Dutch, French Silver, Havana and Tan breeds older than 4 years of age have a 50–80% incidence of uterine adenocarcinoma. Metastases to local tissues, lungs, liver, brain and bones may occur within 1–2 years.

## CASE 208

**What techniques and preparations can be used to administer oral nutritional support in the rabbit?** Most rabbits will tolerate syringe feeding (208) with a liquid food. The recommended intake is 50 ml/kg body weight divided into 3–5 meals per day. The rabbit's normal extruded or pelleted food can be ground down to a powder and then mixed with water to form a paste suitable for syringe feeding. High-fibre (>21%) syringe fed products that are highly palatable and well tolerated by rabbits are also available commercially. These are mixed 1:1.5 with water and any

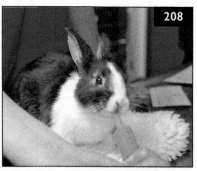

remaining formula may be refrigerated for 48 hours. In rare cases where syringe feeding is not tolerated, placement of a nasogastric or even oesophagostomy tube may prove necessary, and 'fine-grind' products are available which pass more easily through the narrow diameter of these tubes. Oral nutritional support provides calories, nutrients, electrolytes and fluids and is essential in any debilitated rabbit to avoid the onset of ketoacidosis and hepatic lipidosis as a result of fat mobilization, particularly in obese animals. It also helps to rehydrate stomach contents and stimulates normal GI motility, preventing ileus and impactions from developing.

## CASE 209
**What are your main differential diagnoses for splenomegaly in this rabbit?**

- Yersiniosis. *Yersinia pseudotuberculosis* infection is contracted by ingestion of food and bedding contaminated with infected wild rodent and bird droppings. Unwashed plants may also be a source. Clinical signs are non-specific and include weight loss and cachexia. Diagnosis in the live animal is generally not possible. At postmortem examination an enlarged spleen with necrotic foci is apparent. Similar foci may be seen in the lymphoid tissue, especially around the ileocaecocolic junction, and this enlargement may also be palpable in the live animal. Yersiniosis is zoonotic.
- Salmonellosis. The spleen may be grossly enlarged in acute salmonellosis, contracted from ingestion of contaminated food or bedding, again usually from infected wild bird or rodent droppings. Salmonellosis is zoonotic.
- Toxoplasmosis. Acute toxoplasmosis is associated with splenomegaly. *Toxoplasma gondii* oocysts are ingested via food contaminated with infected cat faeces. Other clinical signs seen with acute infection include neurological symptoms (tremors, muscle weakness, paralysis), fever, anorexia and depression.
- Splenic neoplasia.
- Splenic abscess.

## CASE 210
**1 What is your diagnosis?** Ventricular tachycardia with paroxysmal, uniform complexes. Two p waves are seen occurring before the first two QRS complexes, but they have no fixed relationship. The QRS complexes are wide and bizarre and originate from the ventricles.

**2 How would you treat this condition?** Treatment is required as the rabbit is exhibiting clinical signs of compromised cardiac output. In undisturbed rabbits, normal resting heart rates of 140–180 bpm have been recorded; however, in stressed animals in the consulting room, 'normal' heart rate ranges from 180–300 bpm. The underlying rate of the rhythm disturbance is within the normal heart rate range but is too fast for a ventricular rate. The disturbance is relatively frequent and lasts more than four beats. Antiarrhythmic therapy is required in most patients with ventricular tachycardia, as it can progress to ventricular fibrillation and sudden death. Treatment for arrhythmias in pet rabbits has not been reported; however, treatment protocols described for cats may be useful.

## CASE 211
**1 What differential diagnoses are there for an intestinal mass?** Primary neoplasia (e.g. uterine or intestinal); metastatic neoplasia; pyometra; intestinal foreign body with impaction; intussusception; abscessation.

221

**2 What further investigative techniques would you use to reach a diagnosis?**
Radiography of the abdomen and thorax to assess for metastases (including contrast radiography); ultrasonography, although with tympany and the presence of gas this imaging technique may be less informative; haematology and biochemistry may be useful in assessing signs of infection or organ dysfunction.

**3 Describe the management of this case.** The acute onset of gastric and small intestinal dilation and severe hyperglycaemia indicates the need for prompt surgical intervention. It is necessary to provide supportive care for the patient before and during investigative procedures. The rabbit should receive i/v fluids and analgesia before an exploratory laparotomy is performed. Temporary relief of gastric dilation may be

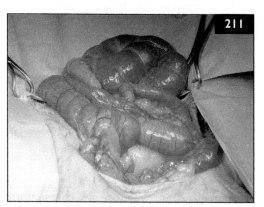

achieved by passing a stomach tube. A caecal intussusception was confirmed in this case (**211**). Resection of the terminal caecum and anastomosis was performed, with careful handling of tissues to prevent shock and ileus. Fluids, analgesia, gut motility stimulants and supplementary feeding were provided during recovery. The prognosis is guarded in cases involving major GI surgery in rabbits.

## CASE 212

**1 What are these structures in the inguinal region (212)?** These are the paired, pouch-like inguinal scent glands. It is normal for them to be filled with a dark waxy secretion.

**2 Where are similar structures also found in the rabbit, and what is their purpose?**
Rabbits also possess chin glands, which are specialized submandibular glands opening on to the underside of the chin, and anal glands. All produce oily secretions containing pheromones that are used for scent marking of the environment and other rabbits. Does mark their kits with chin and inguinal gland secretions to identify them and will be hostile to other young that are not their own. Faeces are an important component of territorial marking and are coated with pheromones produced from the anal glands. Studies have shown that, in the wild, both bucks and does, when on their own territory and surrounded by their own odour and that of their group, win two-thirds of aggressive encounters with other rabbits.

**3 How do they differ between the sexes?** The size of the glands and the degree of marking are androgen-dependent and related to the rabbit's level of sexual activity. Bucks mark more frequently than does, and dominant individuals of both sexes mark more frequently than subordinates. In neutered individuals, marking is reduced but not absent.

## CASE 213

**Evaluate this housing arrangement for a rabbit, noting the important features and their relevance.** Essential features:

- Permanent enclosures provide a natural territory in which the rabbit will feel secure. The rabbit may be difficult to catch in this enclosure. Regular daily handling from a young age will help tame the rabbit and some can be trained to return to the hutch for food rewards.
- High fence to prevent escape by jumping. However, predators may be able to gain access.
- Hutch consisting of solid-fronted compartment for security and warmth, and mesh- fronted compartment allowing ventilation. Hutch is raised to prevent damp and has a sloped felted roof to allow water run-off. It is, however, in an open location with no direct shelter from severe conditions, so it would not be suitable for permanent winter accommodation in temperate climates. Area under the hutch provides shade, as rabbits are prone to heat stress. Rabbit can be secured in hutch at night.
- Good area of natural grazing and exercise space, essential for digestive health and prevention of obesity and musculoskeletal problems. Access to natural daylight and fresh air also beneficial for vitamin D production and prevention of respiratory disease.
- Opportunity to dig, a natural behaviour, but this could result in escape.
- Permanent enclosure, if overstocked, could lead to build-up of coccidial parasites.
- Several 'bolt-holes' to provide secure areas for rabbit to hide or retreat from companions.
- Supply of fresh drinking water via sipper bottle – prevents contamination.

## CASE 214

**1 What are your differential diagnoses?** Uterine neoplasia (e.g. adenocarcinoma), uterine polyps, gravid uterus, endometrial venous aneurysm, pyometra, hydrometra, gravidity.

**2 How would you manage this case?** An exploratory laparotomy should be performed, with ovariohysterectomy if indicated. In this case both uterine horns were found to be enlarged, with evidence of local invasion to the peritoneum. The owner opted for euthanasia at this stage. A diagnosis of uterine adenocarcinoma

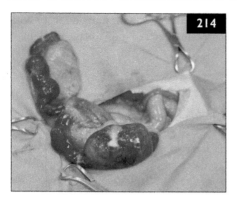

was confirmed on postmortem and histological examination (**214**). This is the most common tumour type in entire adult female rabbits, affecting 60% of does over 4 years of age, with Dutch rabbits being more susceptible. Metastatic spread is common, often locally to other abdominal organs, but also to distant sites via haematogenous spread.

**3 What is the prognosis?** The prognosis is extremely poor if secondary metastases have occurred. Thoracic radiographs should be taken routinely prior to surgery to assess for evidence of metastatic spread to the lungs. Metastatic disease and local peritoneal invasion may not be grossly evident at the time of surgery and the prognosis in any confirmed case of uterine adenocarcinoma should always be guarded. Thoracic radiographs should be repeated six monthly for up to a year post surgery to monitor for pulmonary metastases.

## CASE 215

**What could be the possible behavioural causes of this problem, and how can they be addressed?** There are several medical conditions that can cause a rabbit to toilet in inappropriate areas and it is important that these have been investigated and eliminated before the problem is considered to be behavioural in nature.

Rabbits can easily be trained to use a litter tray due to their tendency to toilet in one area. A breakdown in toilet training can occur in response to litter tray aversion, a change of substrate, problems associated with social relationships within the home and marking behaviour. It is quite common for rabbits to lose all notion of toilet training as they reach puberty; this is often improved with castration. In cases where rabbits feel that they are not safe while using the tray, they may choose to urinate and defecate in an area that appears to be more secure. Occasionally, these areas can be associated with the owner's smell and provide comfort to the rabbit. Owners should ensure that the litter tray is placed in a quiet, secure area, and they must not change the type of litter that they are using. To do so may break the association between the act of elimination and the substrate, leading to a breakdown in basic toilet training. Many toileting problems are caused by overmarking, so once any underlying medical problems have been eliminated, the owner must ensure that any 'accidents' are cleaned using an enzymatic cleaner such as a warm solution of biological washing powder. Faeces and urine can be used to mark boundaries within the territory; a sofa provides a nice high area to promote maximum olfactory impact. Rabbits that routinely mark furniture may be living in a home where they feel less than secure. With time, however, a learned pattern of behaviour may also develop and the rabbit will need to be confined in an area large enough to include its tray for a period of time sufficient to reintroduce the tray.

## CASE 216

**What provisions should be made for their accommodation, to ensure their safety and to minimize mess and damage to the house?** House rabbits must be provided with a secure, large cage or pen where they can retreat to if they desire, and where they can be confined during periods when the owner is not present. Exercise pens manufactured for puppies are a useful method of confining house rabbits safely. These are made of wire panels and can be made into a variety of shapes and sizes. The cage or pen can be lined with synthetic sheepskin, blankets or newspaper, rather than shavings or straw, to minimize mess. Pelleted bedding made out of recycled paper is also useful. A litter tray filled with wood shavings, shredded paper, wood or paper-based cat litter should be provided and cleaned daily. A box or hide area should also be provided. Rabbits are naturally curious and can be very destructive to furniture and fittings. Electrical cables should be covered or taped out of the way. Wallpaper may need to be covered with Perspex at low level to prevent the rabbit stripping it. Carpet may be chewed and can cause gastrointestinal obstructions in the rabbit. Toxic houseplants should be removed (e.g. *Dieffenbachia*, plants grown from bulbs). Access to old painted woodwork should be restricted due to the risk of ingestion of lead-based paint. Other potentially toxic household items include lead curtain weights, linoleum, window putty and foil from wine bottles (all of which may contain lead). Old blankets or rugs can be provided for the rabbit to dig in and minimize the risk of carpets or vinyl flooring being damaged. Hay should always be available *ad libitum*, and feeding from a rack or net will minimize mess. Although they frequently tolerate other pets such as cats and dogs, and sometimes form strong bonds, rabbits should never be left unsupervised with potential predators. Rabbits should always be housed with at least one other rabbit as they are highly social in nature.

## CASE 217

**What advice can you give to facilitate the administration of an oral medication?** Where possible, commercially available liquid preparations should be prescribed, since crushing pills or adding them to food may affect absorption of the drug. If these are not available, oral medication is best given in a suspension, as rabbits do not swallow pills easily. If necessary, pills can be crushed in water or a commercially

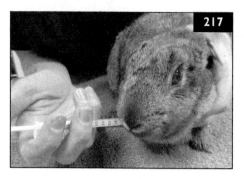

available nutritional supplement and then syringe fed to the rabbit. The tip of the syringe is inserted into the diastema caudal to the incisors (**217**). Rabbits often resist restraint, making it difficult to administer oral medications single-handed. If this is the case, the rabbit may be restrained by wrapping it in a large towel.

## CASE 218

**What normal anatomical features can be seen?** The lateral thoracic view optimizes visualization of the heart, lung fields and thoracic skeleton. Rabbits have a relatively small thoracic cavity in relation to the abdominal cavity and breathing is mainly diaphragmatic. Assessment of the cranial thorax is difficult due to superimposition of the scapulae and muscles of the forelimbs and the small size of the cranial lung fields. Large amounts of intrathoracic fat are often present. The thymus remains large in the adult rabbit and lies ventral to the heart, extending into the thoracic inlet. The heart is relatively small and lies cranially in the thoracic cavity.

The trachea, carina, aorta, caudal lung fields and diaphragm are also visible on the lateral thoracic radiographic view.

## CASE 219

**1 What examination technique is being shown (219)?** Abdominal ballottement. This may be carried out as part of a routine clinical examination and in cases of intestinal ileus to detect caecal resonance.

**2 What conditions may be diagnosed using this technique?** In a normal rabbit, fed a high-fibre diet, the area of resonance should extend over the right epigastric area on the cranioventral right-hand side of the abdomen. Animals fed a high-starch diet, which is rapidly fermented, often have a larger area of resonance extending over both sides of the cranioventral abdomen. In sick animals, or in animals with GI disease where there is an increase in fluid content of the caecum, the resonance is reduced. In obese animals the sound may be more muffled and this should be taken into account. Enlargement of one or more of the abdominal organs will result in displacement of the resonant area. In cases presenting with ileus, more generalized resonance may be found.

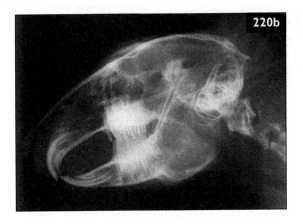

## CASE 220

Describe how this is carried out and in what circumstances it is indicated. A contrast study of the nasolacrimal duct. Pre-contrast plain radiographs should first be taken. Approximately 1 ml of iodine-based contrast material is then instilled into the lacrimal punctum and radiographs of the skull are taken. This technique is extremely useful in evaluating cases of chronic dachryocystitis, where it helps determine whether tooth root changes are an underlying problem. For comparison, (220b) shows the same animal prior to injection of the contrast medium.

## CASE 221

**1 What organism is most likely to be causing the clinical signs and lesions?** *Psoroptes cuniculi*, the rabbit ear mite (221b).

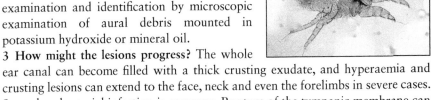

**2 How would you confirm your diagnosis?** Visualization of the mite on otoscopic examination and identification by microscopic examination of aural debris mounted in potassium hydroxide or mineral oil.

**3 How might the lesions progress?** The whole ear canal can become filled with a thick crusting exudate, and hyperaemia and crusting lesions can extend to the face, neck and even the forelimbs in severe cases. Secondary bacterial infection is common. Rupture of the tympanic membrane can occur, leading to an otitis media/interna with associated clinical signs such as head tilt.

**4 What treatment is appropriate?** Ivermectin (0.2–0.4 mg/kg s/c every 10–14 days for 3 doses; selamectin (8–16 mg/kg topically once); moxidectin (0.2 mg/kg s/c every 10 days for 2 doses). Crusts will resolve with treatment but may be softened

227

with mineral oil or petroleum jelly. Resist pulling away scabs and instead allow them to heal and be removed naturally. NSAIDs such as meloxicam (0.3–0.6 mg/kg s/c or p/o) or carprofen (2–4 mg/kg s/c or p/o) are indicated for analgesia and to reduce inflammation. The claws on the hindlimbs should be trimmed to reduce the amount of self-trauma from scratching.

## CASE 222

**1 What disease is shown in the histological section (222)?** Sebaceous adenitis. The section shows a mural infiltrative lymphocytic folliculitis and absence of sebaceous glands. The aetiology is unknown.

**2 What treatment may be attempted?** Treatment with essential fatty acids, retinoids and topical oil soaks or sprays can be attempted but may be unsuccessful.

## CASE 223

**1 What is your diagnosis?** Hypercalciuria and cystic calculi present as radiodense material in the bladder on radiography, and it may be difficult to distinguish between the two.

**2 What further diagnostic tests would you perform?** Ultrasonographic examination will differentiate between discrete calculi and 'sludge' material. Urinalysis should be performed on a sterile sample obtained by cystocentesis or catheterization to rule out underlying bacterial or fungal infections. A complete blood count and serum biochemical assay should also be performed to assess renal function.

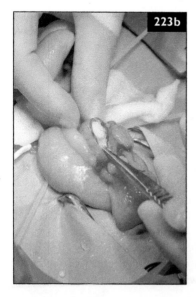

**3 What treatment is indicated?** Cystotomy and removal of thick sludge or a bladder stone is indicated in cases of cystic calculus (223b). This is the treatment of choice for large cystic calculi in the rabbit. Smaller calculi and crystalluria may sometimes be treated by catheterization of the bladder under sedation and careful flushing with saline.

The rabbit should be thoroughly hydrated prior to surgical removal. Analgesics and anti-inflammatory drugs are indicated and should be continued until the rabbit urinates normally. Intravenous fluid therapy should be continued postoperatively and the rabbit should be hospitalized until urination returns to normal.

Antibiotics should be given for 4–6 weeks in cases with concurrent bacterial cystitis.

**4 What preventive measures would you instigate?** Preventive measures include increasing exercise, increasing water intake and reducing dietary calcium intake. Treatment is aimed at reducing calcium levels and increasing urine output. Alfalfa hay and rabbit pellets contain high levels of calcium and should be avoided.

Water intake should be carefully monitored to ensure that the water source is being used. Water intake can be promoted with the provision of both a bowl and a bottle, with rabbits showing a natural preference for bowl drinking.

Analgesics and antibiotics are indicated, but urinary acidifiers are not effective in rabbits.

The rabbit should be encouraged to exercise to ensure normal urination patterns and, if obese, lose weight.

## CASE 224

**What volume of blood constitutes a critical blood loss in a rabbit undergoing a surgical procedure (224)?** Critical blood loss levels in rabbits are 20–30% of circulating blood volume. Total blood volume in a healthy rabbit is calculated as between 5.5% and 7% of body weight. In a 2 kg rabbit, therefore, the total blood volume might be 140 ml and a blood loss of between 28 ml and 42 ml would be critical.

## CASE 225

**Describe your findings and possible treatment options.** A right mandibular fracture is present. There is rostral and lateral displacement of the caudal half of the right mandible resulting in mandibular shortening. There appears to be good alignment of the molars.

If the fracture is stable, healing by callus formation may be acceptable, but the rabbit may require the placement of a nasogastric feeding tube until it is able to masticate normally. If the fracture is unstable, fixation with a bone plate is possible but would be technically challenging.

This rabbit was managed conservatively and required 10 days' hospitalization and supportive care before returning to normal demeanour and appetite.

## CASE 226

**1 Describe what this device is and how it works.** A supraglottic airway device (also referred to as a laryngeal mask) is a soft, non-inflatable, anatomically shaped cuff that is inserted in the mouth and advanced caudally over the glottis. When in the

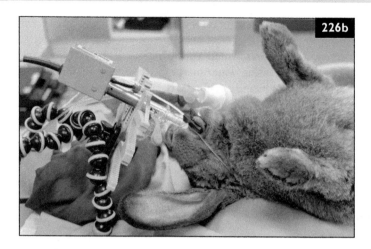

correct position, it creates a seal over the pharyngeal, laryngeal, perilaryngeal and the upper esophageal structures. It is used to deliver inhalation anaesthetic gas to an anaesthetized patient (**226b**).

2 **What are the advantages and disadvantages of supraglottic airway devices?**
*Advantages* of supraglottic airway devices:
- Easy to place, with insertion time of 5–20 seconds.
- Easy to use in an emergency situation.
- No risk of trauma to the lining of the trachea.
- Autoclave compatible.

*Disadvantages* of supraglottic airway devices:
- Expensive in comparison to an endotracheal tube.
- When repositioning the patient, there is a risk that the mask could dislodge from the correct position over the larynx.
- Capnography is required to ensure continued correct placement.
- Any unnoticed food in the mouth could be scooped up into the device and could potentially lead to aspiration or obstruction.

## CASE 227

**Describe how you would collect a sample using a bronchoalveolar lavage technique.**

1 The rabbit is anaesthetized and intubated with a sterile endotracheal tube.
2 The rabbit is positioned in lateral recumbency. If unilateral lung disease is present, the affected lung should be against the table.
3 Ideally, the catheter is pre-measured alongside the rabbit prior to the procedure to gauge the distance needed to advance.

4 A sterile urinary catheter is placed through the ET tube and gently advanced until there is resistance (usually at the point of the bifurcation).

5 Sterile saline (1 ml/kg) is instilled through the endotracheal tube and immediately suctioned using a syringe to collect fluid. Approximately half the total fluid volume instilled should be aspirated back.

6 Samples should be collected in sterile tubes and EDTA for analysis.

## CASE 228

**Is this a treatment you would recommend to owners?** The use of enzymatic products (e.g. papain) to digest trichobezoars is controversial: these products do not actually digest hair (keratin) but may help to break down the matrix holding the material together. Pineapple juice is high in simple sugars, which may lead to caecal dysbiosis and clostridial overgrowth. The perceived beneficial effects of pineapple juice are anecdotal.

For prevention of hair-related problems, the owner should be advised to perform regular grooming of the rabbit. Many perceived hairball-related problems are in fact due to gastric stasis as a result of normal gastric content – which contains ingested hair – that has become dehydrated. If treatment is required, fluid therapy is of most benefit to rehydrate gastric content.

For these reasons, pineapple juice is not a recommended treatment for trichobezoars in rabbits.

## CASE 229

**1 Discuss the thoracic radiographic findings.** There is a diffuse alveolar and interstitial pulmonary pattern with secondary pleural effusion. The visible lung field has generalized ill-defined areas of increased radiopacity with occasional pulmonary nodules. There is border effacement of the cardiac silhouette and dorsal displacement of the trachea.

**2 Based on the radiographic findings, what procedure would be beneficial to the patient?** Further diagnostic tests should ideally be performed to ascertain the cause of the pleural effusion. To alleviate respiratory distress, drainage of the thorax by thoracocentesis under ultrasound guidance should be performed. The rabbit should either be sedated or undergo a local anaesthetic block of the intercostal spaces to facilitate this. Once obtained, cytology can be performed on the sample for evidence of infection or neoplasia.

**3 What is the likely prognosis in this case?** With the degree of pleural effusion and pulmonary nodules, the prognosis in this case would be guarded and neoplasia would be strongly suspected.

## CASE 230

**1 What are these lesions?** The lesions are chalezia or lipid granulomas. They arise from cystic changes to the meibomian gland, thought to arise from irritation of the epithelial lining.

**2 What treatment would you advise to the owner?** If the rabbit is asymptomatic and the chalezia are not causing deviation of the eyelid or trauma to the corneal surface, no treatment is required. If they are problematic, removal by curettage should be performed. This is often achievable without sedation using local anaesthetic eye drops.

## CASE 231

**1 Discuss the findings from this rostral cross-section image taken at the level of the upper incisors.** The right rostral nasal cavity displays complete atrophy of the ventral nasal conchae. This is particularly obvious when compared to the contralateral side.

The right maxillary sinus is filled with fluid. There is no deviation of the nasal septum and no destruction of the surrounding bone. The incisors appear symmetrical and grossly normal at this level.

**2 What is your diagnosis?** The diagnosis is a severe atrophic rhinosinusitis. The most likely aetiology is bacterial infection. Swabs of the right nasal passage should be obtained and bacterial and fungal cultures performed to determine the causative agent.

## CASE 232

**Describe the changes seen at the level of the tympanic bulla (232b).** The left tympanic bulla is gas-filled and appears grossly normal at this level of cross section.

The right tympanic bulla is ill-defined and filled with soft tissue dense material with subtle areas of mineralized foci. There is marked lysis of the ventral osseous margin of the bulla and general bone thinning when compared to the opposite side.

A round, soft tissue mass is present lateral to the right tympanic bulla. This mass is filled with a mixture of soft tissue and mineralized structures.

The rabbit appears to have advanced otitis media with localized bone destruction and abscess formation. From this cross-sectional image, neoplasia cannot be ruled out, although advanced infection is most likely.

# Index

**Note:** References are to page numbers

# Index

# Index

## Also available in the Self-Assessment Color Review series